This book is dedicated to all patients with pancreatic cancer and their family and friends. You are the most courageous and determined patients who amaze and humble us every day. This life-altering journey is a profound experience for you and those who love you. We are most grateful for the opportunity to care for such a special group of patients.

JoAnn Coleman and Nita Ahuja

CONTENTS

Contributors

Marian Grant, DNP, CRNP, ACHPN
Assistant Professor
University of Maryland School of Nursing
Baltimore, MD

Gary R. Shapiro, MD
Chairman, Department of Oncology
Johns Hopkins Bayview Medical Center
Director, Johns Hopkins Geriatric Oncology Program
The Sidney Kimmel Comprehensive Cancer Center at
    Johns Hopkins
Baltimore, MD

Ella-Mae Shupe, RN
Nurse Clinician
Oncology Ambulatory Services
The Sidney Kimmel Comprehensive Cancer Center at
    Johns Hopkins
Baltimore, MD

PREFACE

Receiving a diagnosis of pancreatic cancer is overwhelming. Trying to determine your next steps following the diagnosis can be equally paralyzing. Rather than entering an environment that is totally foreign to you, consider learning some information in advance.

This book is part of a series of *Johns Hopkins Medicine Cancer Patients' Guides* designed to educate newly diagnosed patients about their cancer diagnosis and the treatments that may lie ahead. This information is provided to help guide you and your support teams of family, friends, and healthcare providers from the time cancer is confirmed to the time treatment is completed.

Don't feel the need to read the entire book at once. It is intended for you to read at your leisure and when you feel ready for additional information. Resource information, including access to Johns Hopkins oncology specialists, is also contained within these pages.

Until there is a cure and there are effective ways to prevent pancreatic cancer, the entire Johns Hopkins medical team is committed to quality, compassionate, and comprehensive care of patients with this cancer.

Introduction

How to Use This Book to Your Benefit

Y ou will receive a lot of information from your health-care team. You will also probably seek some out on the Internet or in bookstores. No doubt friends and family members, meaning well, will offer you advice on what to do and when to do it, and will try to steer you in certain directions. Try to relax. You have heard words you wish you had never heard said about you—that you have pancreatic cancer. Even after hearing such news, it is important to take the time to empower yourself with accurate information so that you can participate in the decision making about your care and treatment.

This book is designed to be a how-to guide that will take you through the maze of treatment options, and at times, complicated schedules. It will help you to put together a plan of action so that you can become a cancer survivor. While not all patients with pancreatic cancer can be cured, many are living active lives and managing their disease. For those less fortunate, in whom the cancer is not cured, this book also offers strength and guidance. Many researchers and clinicians are committed to finding better treatments with the goal of finding a cure for pancreatic cancer.

This book is broken down into chapters and includes an index in the back as well as credible resources listed for your further review and education. By empowering yourself with accurate, understandable information, you are in a much better position to make treatment decisions.

There is a natural sense of urgency to proceed with some type of treatment as soon as possible when you have a diagnosis of pancreatic cancer. However, the initial decision you make about where to receive treatment and from which multidisciplinary team can be crucial in determining the overall treatment outcome. This book will give you the information and tools you need to make informed decisions.

The majority of the tumors of the pancreas are pancreatic adenocarcinomas. Other rarer forms of pancreas tumors are termed endocrine tumors of the pancreas. This book will focus primarily on diagnosis and treatment of adenocarcinomas of the pancreas, unless otherwise stated. Endocrine tumors are rare cancers and may have different signs and symptoms. These tumors are diagnosed by different tests, treatment methods, and prognoses. For more information on endocrine tumors of the pancreas, please refer to the National Cancer Institute–Designated Comprehensive Cancer Centers at http://www.cancer.gov/.

Let's begin now with understanding what has happened and what the steps are to get you well again.

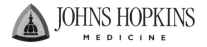

First Steps—
I've Been Diagnosed with
Pancreatic Cancer

Y ou have recently been told that you have a mass in your pancreas and that this pancreatic mass may be cancer, or you have had a biopsy of a mass in your pancreas that has been diagnosed as cancer of the pancreas. No doubt you may be in shock after hearing these words. Some patients think "I don't have a family history of any pancreatic issues, so how is this possible? I don't have any risk factors, so how did I get this cancer? I have regular health checkups, so why do I have pancreatic cancer?" Let's begin by answering these common questions.

Only 10% of people diagnosed with pancreatic cancer have a family history, meaning 90% of the people diagnosed with pancreatic cancer have no family history at all. Sometimes people assume that any type of cancer in the family is the same as having a history of pancreatic cancer in the family, but this isn't true. According to the American Cancer Society, about one in three people in the United States will develop some type of cancer in their lifetime. In the United States cancer of the pancreas is the fourth leading cause of cancer deaths in both men and women. The incidence of pancreatic cancer has been slowly rising.

By and large, most people who are diagnosed with pancreatic cancer have no family history that predisposes them to getting this disease. However, a history of certain cancers, such as breast, ovarian, melanoma, and pancreatic cancers, seen in a number of family members would raise concern about a potential genetic link, and talking with a genetic counselor may be recommended.

WHERE IS THE PANCREAS?

The pancreas is an organ of the digestive system. It is about 6 inches long, located deep in the abdomen behind the stomach and in front of your backbone. The pancreas is shaped like a pear sitting on its side (see Figure 1). The wide end of the pancreas, called the head, lies in the right middle side of your abdomen tucked into the first part of your small bowel (the duodenum). The middle sections of the pancreas are called the neck and body and are tucked behind the stomach. The thin end is the tail of the pancreas and is located on the left side of the abdomen next to the spleen. The uncinate process is the part of the gland that lies behind and under the head of the pancreas. There is a large main pancreatic duct, or passage, that runs through the middle of the pancreas. The pancreatic juices collect in the pancreas and travel through the duct into the duodenum, where they then help break down fats and other foods to keep your body working.

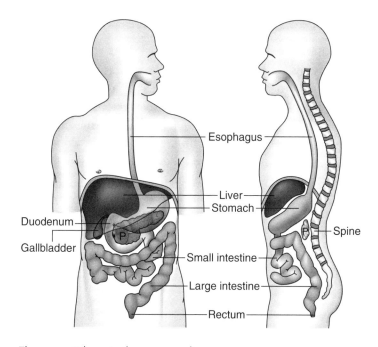

Figure 1   Where is the pancreas?

Adapted from artwork by Jennifer Parsons Brumbaugh from http://pathology. jhu.edu/pancreas.

Another important passage is the common bile duct, which comes from the gallbladder to the back of the head of the pancreas to a place where it joins the main pancreatic duct and forms an opening into the duodenum called the ampulla of Vater. This is where the bile that is made in your liver travels down the common bile duct and out into the duodenum to also help with digesting your food.

Two important blood vessels associated with the pancreas are the superior mesenteric artery and the superior mesenteric vein, which are found behind the neck of the pancreas and in front of the uncinate process.

WHAT DOES THE PANCREAS DO IN THE BODY?

The pancreas has two main functions because there are two types of cells that make up the pancreas. The exocrine cells make up about 95% of the pancreas and produce enzymes that help break down food—the exocrine function of the pancreas. The main pancreatic duct empties the enzymes into the duodenum, where the enzymes break down fats and other foods to keep your body working. The endocrine cells of the pancreas, called the islets of Langerhans, make up the other 5% of the pancreas and produce hormones that are released into the bloodstream. The two main endocrine hormones are insulin and glucagon, which help to keep the proper level of sugar in your blood and perform the endocrine function of the pancreas. So, tumors arising in the endocrine cells of the pancreas are called neuroendocrine tumors, or pancreas endocrine tumors.

TYPES OF PANCREATIC CANCER

The most common types of pancreatic cancer are exocrine tumors, called adenocarcinomas, in which the cancer cells start in the lining of the pancreatic duct and continue to grow within the pancreas. About two-thirds of all pancreatic cancers form in the head of the pancreas; the other third form in the body and tail of the pancreas. These tumors are malignant, or cancerous, and can spread into nearby tissues and organs. The cancerous pancreatic cells can also travel through the blood and lymphatic system to other parts of the body. When cancer cells leave the pancreas and spread to other parts of the body, it is called a metastatic cancer. Although the overwhelming majority of exocrine tumors of the pancreas are adenocarcinomas, there are other rare types. These are listed here:

Acinar cell carcinoma

Adenosquamous carcinoma

Pancreatoblastoma

Cystic tumors

> Mucinous cystic tumors
>
> Serous cystic tumors
>
> Solid and pseudopapillary tumors
>
> Intraductal papillary mucinous neoplasms (IPMNs)

Tumors also can be found in the endocrine cells of the pancreas, although pancreas endocrine tumors are rare. These tumors may be benign or malignant and tend to be slow growing. These tumors are grouped as functional (they produce hormones) or nonfunctional (they do not produce hormones). Most of the functional endocrine tumors are benign. However, 90% of the nonfunctional endocrine tumors of the pancreas are malignant or cancerous. Other rare forms of pancreatic endocrine cancer are listed here:

Gastrinomas (Zollinger-Ellison syndrome)

Glucagonomas

Insulinomas

Somatostatinomas

VIPomas (vasoactive intestinal peptide-releasing tumor, or Verner-Morrison syndrome)

Multiple endocrinc neoplasia type I (MENI)

Endocrine tumors of the pancreas are rare cancers, may have different signs and symptoms, are diagnosed by different tests, and have different treatment and prognoses. The remainder of the book will focus on diagnosis and treatment of adenocarcinomas of the pancreas, unless otherwise stated. For more information on endocrine tumors of the pancreas, please refer to the Web site of the National Cancer Institute—Designated Comprehensive Cancer Centers at http://www.cancer.gov/.

RISK FACTORS

No one knows the exact cause or causes of pancreatic cancer. There are a number of risk factors that may increase the likelihood that a person will develop pancreatic cancer. Smoking is the most significant risk factor known and appears to cause 25% of all cases of pancreatic cancer. A person who smokes cigarettes is twice as likely to develop pancreatic cancer than a person who does not. Most people who are diagnosed with pancreatic cancer are over the age of 60, so the chance of developing pancreatic cancer increases with age. A person who has one first-degree relative (mother, father, brother, sister, or child) with pancreatic cancer has a two to three times increased risk of developing this cancer compared with people with no family history. A person is at greater risk of developing pancreatic cancer as the number of family members affected with pancreatic cancer increases.

The risk of pancreatic cancer is greater when there is a history of familial breast cancer, especially if the person has a defect in a gene called BRCA2. The risk of pancreatic cancer is even higher in persons with certain other hereditary syndromes, such as hereditary pancreatitis, multiple endocrine neoplasia, hereditary nonpolyposis colorectal cancer, familial adenomatous polyposis and Gardner syndrome, familial atypical multiple mole melanoma syndrome, and

Von Hippel-Lindau syndrome. Moreover, a history of colon cancer or familial melanoma increases a person's risk for pancreatic cancer. A person who smokes and has a family history of pancreatic cancer has an increased risk of developing pancreatic cancer up to 10 years earlier than his or her diagnosed family members.

People with chronic pancreatitis have an increased risk of developing pancreatic cancer, especially if they were diagnosed with pancreatitis at a young age. Chronic pancreatitis is usually diagnosed in persons aged 35 to 45 years and mostly in persons who drink large amounts of alcohol over many years. Other causes of chronic pancreatitis, such as mumps and autoimmune diseases, may also lead to pancreatic cancer. African Americans have a higher occurrence of pancreatic cancer compared with other races. Persons of Ashkenazi Jewish ancestry also have a higher occurrence of pancreatic cancer. Men are diagnosed with pancreatic cancer at a slightly higher rate than women. Persons with diabetes are also twice as likely to be diagnosed with pancreatic cancer. It is not clear whether diabetes plays a role in the development of pancreatic cancer or whether precancerous cells cause diabetes.

The development of pancreatic cancer and its relationship to a person's diet is not clear. It is thought that a diet high in red meats, animal fats, processed meats, and carbohydrates increases the risk of developing pancreatic cancer. Other foods that may be a risk associated with the development of pancreatic cancer are meats that are very well cooked, especially charred meats; foods high in salt and refined sugars; or foods that have been smoked, dehydrated, or fried. A significant increased risk for developing pancreatic cancer is seen in persons who are considered clinically obese (20% or more over an individual's ideal body weight). Finally, a large population study found that lack of physical activity or exercise was associated with an increased risk of pancreatic cancer.

HOW PANCREATIC CANCERS ARE FOUND AND IDENTIFIED

The initial symptoms of pancreatic cancer are not always obvious; they can be subtle and usually develop over time. Early pancreatic cancer often has no symptoms, which is why for many people the pancreatic cancer has often spread by the time they are aware of any signs or symptoms or it is noticed by a doctor. A person may have different symptoms depending on the location, type, and stage of the cancer. A person may report gradual onset of nonspecific symptoms such as fatigue, weakness, nausea, and abdominal pain in the upper abdomen that spreads around both sides to the back or back pain. Significant weight loss also may be seen when a person has no appetite or is unable to take in nutrients from food when the pancreatic duct is obstructed, causing pancreatic exocrine insufficiency (a decrease in the amount of enzymes made by the pancreas).

These initial symptoms can be easily attributed to other things and also can be caused by other infections, so unless a physician has good reasons to suspect an underlying pancreatic cancer, a delay in diagnosis of pancreatic cancer is common. Less than a third of persons with pancreatic cancer are diagnosed within 2 months of the onset of their symptoms. Pain is the most common presenting symptom in a person with pancreatic cancer. The onset of diabetes within the previous year or two is sometimes also associated with pancreatic cancer.

Pancreatic cancers can occur in various parts of this small gland and can have somewhat different signs. The most common sign of a pancreatic cancer in the head of the pancreas is yellow eyes and skin, also known as painless obstructive jaundice. This is caused by the cancer blocking the bile duct where the duct enters the pancreas. People with this sign may see their physician before the cancer grows large enough to cause abdominal pain. People usually notice a darkening of their urine and a lighter color to their bowel movements. Subtle to uncontrolled itching, called pruritus, may also occur when a person has obstructive jaundice. Diarrhea in the form of loose, watery, oily, or foul-smelling bowel movements can occur in some people. The diarrhea is caused by a lack of pancreatic enzymes available to help digest foods, particularly foods high in fat. The lack of pancreatic enzymes can be from the pancreas not being able to make enough enzymes or from a blockage in the pancreas not allowing the enzymes to reach the small bowel to help with digestion.

For pancreatic cancers in the rest of the pancreas gland, known as the body and tail of the pancreas, symptoms that may be seen are indigestion, a decrease in appetite, nausea, subtle weight loss, and back pain. Pain on a person's left side may, along with weight loss, fatigue, and malaise, be a symptom of a cancer in the tail of the pancreas. Depression is reported to be more common in persons with pancreatic cancer than in persons with other abdominal cancers. In some persons, depression may be the most prominent presenting symptom. Blood clots in the legs (deep vein thrombosis) or in the lungs (pulmonary embolism) may also occur with higher frequency in persons with pancreatic cancer. A person with advanced pancreatic cancer may also have ascites (fluid in the abdomen), an enlarged liver from metastatic disease in the liver, or persistent back pain from the pancreatic cancer surrounding important blood vessels and nerves found behind the pancreas.

If a pancreatic cancer is suspected, a number of tests may be performed to help define what is going on in the pancreas. These tests will be done after your physician has asked about your medical and family history and performed a complete physical examination. There is no specific blood test for detecting or diagnosing pancreatic cancer. A person with obstructive jaundice usually has abnormal blood test results, including higher than normal bilirubin, alkaline phosphatase, and gamma-glutamyl transpeptidase (GGT) levels. Other blood test results, such as the levels of pancreatic enzyme (amylase and lipase), are usually not abnormal in pancreatic cancer. A small number (5%) of persons with pancreatic cancer present with acute pancreatitis in which elevated levels of amylase and lipase are seen.

A useful cancer marker for pancreatic cancer is carbohydrate antigen 19-9 (CA 19-9). CA 19-9 antigens are foreign substances released by pancreatic cancer cells, so testing for their presence in the blood can help detect cancers. Testing for CA 19-9 levels has not been proven to be effective for the early detection of small, early-stage pancreatic cancer or as a screening tool. The CA 19-9 level has been shown to be useful as a surveillance marker after the diagnosis of pancreatic cancer is confirmed and if the CA 19-9 level was elevated prior to any treatment. The CA 19-9 level can be used to assess whether there is a response to treatment (in which case the level should decrease) or to monitor for any recurrence or progression of pancreatic cancer (the level should rise). This helps your physician decide whether treatment should be changed or whether additional tests are needed.

Carcinoembryonic antigen (CEA) level is another blood test that measures the level of CEA protein in the blood. CEA is commonly used as a cancer marker in many gastrointestinal cancers. CEA level is not used as a diagnostic screening test for pancreatic cancer because CEA is not made by all pancreatic cancers and because other conditions, such as smoking or other cancers, can cause a rise in the CEA level.

Certain imaging studies provide the best information in the form of pictures of the pancreas and its nearby organs, tissues, blood vessels, and nerves. These studies help to diagnose pancreatic cancer as well as monitor the effects of treatment. A computed tomography (CT) scan with oral (taken by mouth) and intravenous (IV) dye is believed to be the most useful test to detect pancreatic cancer because it can assess the entire abdomen and pelvis. A CT scan is often done to monitor a person after treatment to see whether the cancer has recurred or spread to another area in the abdomen, or whether the cancer has changed in size. Multidetector-row spiral CT (also called helical CT) with three-dimensional pictures is currently the most accurate method to detect pancreatic cancers and gives the best detail to allow for appropriate treatment.

Magnetic resonance imaging (MRI) gives different pictures than a CT scan and may provide different information. MRI does not require contrast dye and may be used for people who are allergic to the dye needed for CT scans. Although these imaging studies may show a suspicious mass in the pancreas, the gold standard for diagnosing pancreatic cancer remains taking a small sample of tissue (biopsy) from the mass to be looked at under a microscope by a pathologist to see what type of pancreatic cancer exists.

Endoscopic ultrasound (EUS) is a useful procedure to diagnose pancreatic cancer. It is also the best procedure to make a definitive diagnosis of pancreatic cancer. This is done by passing a fine needle (known as a fine needle aspiration, or FNA) into a mass in the pancreas and taking a small sample (biopsy) for a pathologist to look at under a microscope to see if the cells are pancreatic cancer. EUS also helps to determine the size and location of a cancer in the pancreas and whether the cancer has spread to nearby lymph nodes, blood vessels, or other tissues. EUS is currently the best test to find small pancreatic cancers that could not be found by other studies but are suspected based on a patient's history or laboratory tests. EUS is also used to screen persons at high risk for developing pancreatic cancer, because it can find early changes in the pancreas in this particular group.

Endoscopic retrograde cholangiopancreatography (ERCP) is another test to help detect pancreatic cancer when other tests fail or when a person has obstructive jaundice. When the bile duct is blocked by a pancreatic tumor and causes obstructive jaundice, a tube (stent) can be placed into the obstructed bile duct to help keep the bile duct open and allow the free flow of bile into the gastrointestinal tract to aid in digestion during an ERCP. A biopsy or brushing of the tumor to obtain cells may also be done at the time of ERCP to help with diagnosis. Possible risks of ERCP are acute pancreatitis and bleeding into the gastrointestinal tract. Another way to obtain tissue from a suspicious pancreatic mass is to use a CT scan or ultrasound to guide a needle directly through the skin and into the mass (known as an FNA).

Percutaneous transhepatic cholangiography (PTC) is used to take pictures of the bile ducts that drain the liver. A small needle is placed into the liver to reach the bile ducts. Once in the bile duct, a dye is put into the bile duct system and X-ray pictures are taken to look for the site of blockage caused by a pancreatic lesion. A sample of bile can be taken during PTC to look for cancer cells. A small, strawlike tube called a percutaneous biliary drain (PBD) can be placed in the bile duct to allow the free flow of bile. This tube is placed through the skin, into the liver, and into a major bile duct in the liver; it then passes along the bile duct inside the liver into the large bile duct that goes from the liver to the back side of the pancreas and finally ends in the first part of the small bowel (the duodenum).

A positron emission tomography (PET) scan is a special scan that uses a small amount of radioactive glucose (sugar) that is injected into a vein. A special camera looks for the radioactive glucose that has been taken up by cancer cells. A computer then makes a picture to show the location of the cancer cells. Cancer cells take in more glucose than normal cells, so a PET scan can help find cancer cells in the pancreas as well as in other parts of the body. A PET scan can be combined with a CT scan to better detect cancer in the body. Currently, the usefulness of PET scans in pancreatic cancer is still being considered because other conditions or infections may cause a false reading.

Although these tests can be useful in the diagnosis of pancreatic cancer, sometimes a pancreatic cancer may be hard to diagnose with these means. The finding of a mass in the pancreas in a previously healthy patient is considered abnormal and worrisome. If these tests fail to diagnose a pancreatic cancer, a surgeon will then recommend surgery to either biopsy the mass or to remove the mass. Sometimes, in patients who are already known to have pancreatic cancer, a staging laparoscopy is performed. Laparoscopy is surgery that uses a thin, lighted tube (a laparoscope) with a camera inserted through a cut (incision) in the belly to look at the abdominal organs. This procedure may be done to see if the pancreatic cancer has spread (metastasized) throughout the abdomen or to other organs or blood vessels. A piece of the cancer also can be taken through the tube at the time of laparoscopy for biopsy.

HOW TO SELECT YOUR ONCOLOGY TEAM

You want to be in the hands of experts who will provide the best cancer care. You need to obtain care from hospitals or doctors that care for large numbers of people with pancreatic cancer. Do not rely on self-promoting advertisements on television or the Internet as your way to select a facility or doctor. A personal physician, friends, relatives, or neighbors can point you toward the best oncologists and the best cancer centers in your area. Seek an accredited cancer program, as deemed so by the American College of Surgeons, the National Cancer Institute, and the National Comprehensive Cancer Network. Additional information is available from your local medical society, hospital, or medical school. You also can call (800) 4-CANCER to learn about nearby treatment facilities supported by the National Cancer Institute or get a list of qualified doctors through the American Board of Medical Specialties (ABMS) (http://www.abms.org/WC/login.aspx).

Studies have confirmed that being treated by pancreatic cancer specialists give you higher odds of survival than being treated by a general surgeon. If you are referred to a "surgeon for pancreatic cancer," ask questions such as the following:

- How many pancreatic *cancer* surgeries does the surgeon do a year?

- What is his or her mortality rate?

- What is his or her rate of postoperative complications?

- What other types of surgeries does he or she do, and how much of his or her time is spent doing pancreatic cancer surgery? It has been shown that for surgery on the pancreas, the best outcomes (survival after surgery) are at hospitals that perform a high volume (number) of pancreatic surgeries each year (at least 11 pancreatic resections per year, as defined by the Leapfrog group. The Leapfrog group is a coalition of 150 large public and private employers representing more than 40 million people and is aimed at improving healthcare quality.).

- Is the surgeon board certified and in what field or fields?

- How long has the surgeon been in practice?

- Where did the surgeon train and under what surgeon did he or she study?

- Does the surgeon regularly attend pancreatic cancer tumor boards to present cases for team discussion?

- Does the surgeon work with a multidisciplinary team of physicians who also specialize in pancreatic cancer so that continuity of your care can be maintained?

- What is the surgeon's philosophy on educating patients about their treatment options?

These are all questions you have the right to have answered before deciding that this particular doctor should be your pancreatic surgical oncologist. If the surgeon hesitates about answering any of the questions, consider this a sign that the surgeon may not be the one you want to attempt to bond with and to assist you in your fight against your pancreatic cancer.

It is not unusual, in fact it is recommended, to get a second opinion after the first consultation, particularly if you have first been seen at a hospital or physician's office where pancreatic cancer specialists may not be available. The first doctor's assessment may be correct, but you may want the diagnosis confirmed, as well as treatment options reviewed, before starting any course of treatment. Every patient has the right to seek a second opinion.

A number of cancer centers have established multidisciplinary cancer groups focused on the treatment of pancreatic cancers. These clinics are committed to the treatment of pancreatic cancers and will include specialists in surgery, medical oncology, and radiation oncology, as well as a team of nurses. A multidisciplinary focus ensures that you can be seen by multiple specialists simultaneously, that you benefit from their collective wisdom, and that your treatment plan employs all effective modalities of treatments.

GATHERING RECORDS BEFORE THE FIRST VISIT

In preparation for your scheduled visit to see your doctor—whether that is a surgeon, medical oncologist, or radiation oncologist—to determine a plan of treatment for pancreatic cancer, you will need to gather your medical records and information from your current physician. The specific information to have available, either to have sent to the doctor's or clinic's office ahead of time or to bring with you to your appointment, is your current medical history and physical examination; recent imaging studies (CT scan, MRI/ magnetic resonance cholangiopancreatography [MRCP],

ERCP, EUS, any other studies); current blood work, including any tests for cancer markers (CA 19-9, CEA); and original pathology slides (the glass slides with the tissue) from any biopsies related to your diagnosis. For imaging studies, the actual X-ray films or digital copies of the films on a CD are needed, along with the written report. You may need to pick all of these items up and hand-carry them with you to your consultation, or they may be sent in ahead of time upon request.

You may wonder why you need to get these things if the doctor already has the reports. All accredited cancer centers are required to review these images, especially the pathology slides, to make sure the diagnosis of pancreatic cancer is correct. There have been times when a review of the slides by a pathologist who specializes in pancreatic cancer led to a different diagnosis. Accuracy is key for treatment. The same can occur with a review of previous imaging. New imaging or more recent imaging can be compared with previous imaging and may reveal a different picture altogether that would change the treatment plan or diagnosis. Your treatment plan at every step is based on this information being correct.

CANCER STAGING

Once an accurate diagnosis has been made, you must consider treatment options. Treatment options for pancreatic cancer depend on the stage of your disease and your general health. Staging pancreatic cancer is a way of determining the extent of the cancer in your body by looking at the size of the cancer, whether the cancer has spread, and where it has spread. It is important to know the stage of pancreatic cancer because treatment is often decided according to the stage of the cancer. Your doctor may not be able to tell you the exact stage of your cancer until after surgery, if that is the plan of treatment.

The two main ways of staging pancreatic cancer are the TNM system and the stage number system. TNM stands for tumor, node, metastasis. This system describes the size of a primary pancreatic tumor ("T"), whether there are lymph nodes ("N") with cancer cells in them, and whether the cancer has spread, or metastasized ("M"), to a different part of the body.

The "T" is the first part of the TNM classification, and it refers to the size and extent of the tumor. The AJCC 2010 classification for exocrine and endocrine pancreas tumors is detailed here. The lymph node and metastasis status are the same.

- T is (carcinoma in situ) is very early stage pancreatic cancer that has not had a chance to spread. This is uncommon in pancreatic cancer.

- T1 means the size of the tumor in the pancreas is 2 cm or less.

- T2 means the tumor is more than 2 cm in size.

- T3 means the cancer has grown into surrounding tissues around the pancreas but does not involve the celiac nerve or the superior mesenteric artery.

- T4 means the cancer involves the celiac nerve or the superior mesenteric artery.

The "N" refers to lymph nodes. Pancreatic cancer can spread via lymph nodes, so this information is important. The lymph nodes are a part of the lymphatic system (a system similar to the blood vessel system). Often this information will only be available after surgery is done.

- N0 means there are no lymph nodes containing cancer.

- N1 means there are lymph nodes that contain cancer cells and that the cancer has more likely spread further than the pancreas itself. N1 is divided into two substages:

  - N1a—There is cancer in a single nearby lymph node.

  - N1b—There is cancer in more than one lymph node.

The "M" part of the classification refers to whether distant metastases are present.

- M0 means the cancer has not spread into distant organs such as the liver or lungs.

- M1 means the cancer has spread to other organs.

There are five numbered stages of pancreatic cancer, some of which are divided into lettered substages (see Table 1).

Stage 0—This is noninvasive pancreatic cancer, which is rare. The cancer is still "in situ," which means the cancer is still in place (noninvasive) and has no potential of spreading to another organ.

Stage IA—This is the earliest stage of invasive pancreatic cancer. The cancer is completely inside the pancreas and measures 2 cm or less.

Stage IB—The cancer is completely inside the pancreas and measures greater than 2 cm.

Stage IIA—The cancer has started to grow into nearby tissues around the pancreas. It may be in the duodenum or the bile duct. However, there is no cancer inside the nearby lymph nodes, nor does it involve the local major blood vessels (the superior mesenteric artery or celiac axis).

Table 1 Stages of Pancreatic Cancer

Stage Number	Description	TNM Stage	Surgical Resection Category
Stage IA	This is the earliest stage of cancer. The cancer is completely inside the pancreas and measures 2 cm or less.	T1; N0; M0	Resectable/local
Stage IB	The cancer is completely inside the pancreas and measures more than 2 cm.	T2; N0; M0	Resectable/local
Stage IIA	The cancer has started to grow into nearby tissues around the pancreas. It may be in the duodenum or the bile duct, but there is no cancer inside the nearby lymph nodes, nor does it involve the local major blood vessels (superior mesenteric artery or celiac axis).	T3; N0; M0	Potentially resectable/ locally advanced
Stage IIB	The cancer may or may not have spread outside the pancreas but does not involve the celiac axis or superior mesenteric artery. Cancer has spread to local lymph nodes.	T3; N1; M0	Potentially resectable/ locally advanced
Stage III	The primary tumor can be any size and has grown into major arteries, veins, and/or the celiac axis. Cancer may also have spread to nearby lymph nodes.	T1, 2, or 3; N1; M0	Likely unresectable/ locally advanced
Stage IV	The primary tumor may be any size. The cancer has spread to another part of the body such as the liver, abdominal wall, lungs, and/or distant lymph nodes.	Any T; any N; M1	Unresectable/ metastatic

Stage IIB—The cancer may or may not have spread outside the pancreas but does not involve the major blood vessels (the celiac axis or superior mesenteric artery). Cancer has spread to local lymph nodes.

Stage III—The primary tumor can be any size and has grown into major arteries, veins, or the celiac axis. Cancer also may have spread to nearby lymph nodes.

Stage IV—The primary tumor may be any size. The cancer has spread, or metastasized, to another part of the body such as the liver, abdominal wall, lungs, or distant lymph nodes.

CANCER GRADE

The grade of cancer cells may be recorded as part of the pathology report. This can give additional information on how the cancer will behave.

- Well-differentiated—slow-growing cancer cells
- Moderately differentiated—average-growing cancer cells
- Poorly differentiated—rapidly growing cancer cells

UNDERSTANDING THE STAGE AND GRADE

Do not confuse stage with grade! This is a very common mistake. They are very different. Grade is related to cell growth. Stage combines several pieces of information (size of the tumor, node involvement, and other organ or blood vessel involvement) and is in some degree tied to survival estimates. Remember, however, that you are not a statistic. You are an individual person. People fall on both sides of the statistical curve to produce survival statistics. You are embarking on doing whatever you need to do to be on the survival side of the curve.

GENETICS OF PANCREATIC CANCER

Most cancers of the pancreas are caused by a change or mutation in the DNA copying of a cell that causes that cell to grow and divide without any control; this abnormal cell then has the ability to live forever. Changes in DNA can occur all the time, especially when cells divide, but cells can repair changes to their DNA. Sometimes the repair mechanism does not work; when this happens, the change in the DNA is then passed along to future copies of the cell. This, in turn, causes more abnormal cells to be made and continue to grow unchecked, which can then lead to a cancer.

The DNA changes, or mutations, that cause pancreatic cancer can be passed on (inherited) from a parent or they can be acquired. Random changes in a person's DNA or factors in the environment, such as chemical or radiation exposures that occur over a person's lifetime, can lead to acquired changes or mutations that cause a cancer to grow. Scientists are still learning about the complex interactions of genes and other factors that may lead to changes in a cell and the cascade of events that cause a cancer to start and grow. Not everyone who has an acquired change or mutation will develop pancreatic cancer.

Inherited changes or mutations that are passed along in the DNA of a person's reproductive cells can then be passed along to that person's children. When pancreatic cancer is inherited, it is called familial pancreatic cancer because it runs in families. Researchers looking into the development of pancreatic cancer are interested in families with specific inherited genes. As stated before, about 10% of pancreatic cancers are inherited from a parent. Researchers believe that studying specific cancer genes may provide a better understanding of the causes of pancreatic cancer, which may in turn lead to a useful screening tool for this cancer.

Researchers in the United States have set up national pancreatic cancer registries to study the hereditary factors that may influence pancreatic cancer. A listing of several such registries in the United States and internationally is available at http://www.pancreatica.org/registries.html.

The following known hereditary syndromes or disorders are being studied for connections to pancreatic cancer.

Familial breast cancer syndrome. People with the breast cancer 2 gene (*BRCA2*) mutations are known to have an increased risk for several cancers, including pancreatic cancer. A mutation in the *BRCA2* gene is found in approximately 1% of the Ashkenazi Jewish population and is responsible for a ten-fold increased risk of developing pancreatic cancer. A defect in the *BRCA1* gene, which is found in 1.5% of the Ashkenazi Jewish population, leads to a two-fold increased risk for developing pancreatic cancer. Persons who carry the *BRCA2* mutation have a 5% lifetime risk of developing pancreatic cancer.

Cystic fibrosis. The mutation that causes cystic fibrosis (the *CFTR* mutation) affects cells that line the pancreas and causes a decrease in pancreatic enzymes as well as chronic pancreatitis. The risk of developing pancreatic cancer before the age of 60 is two times higher in people with the *CFTR* mutation than in those without it.

Familial adenomatous polyposis (FAP). FAP is a rare hereditary form of colon cancer in which a person develops hundreds to thousands of noncancerous polyps that cover the inside of the colon. The adenomatous polyposis coli (*APC*) gene becomes mutated, and instead of keeping the formation of colon cancer in check, it allows the cancer to grow. The mutated *APC* gene is linked to other cancers, such as pancreatic, thyroid, small bowel, and stomach cancers.

Familial atypical multiple mole melanoma (FAMMM) syndrome. People with FAMMM syndrome have many different-sized skin moles that are irregular in shape and raised from the skin. Persons with this syndrome have a mutation of the *p16* gene and have a 17% risk of developing pancreatic cancer.

Fanconi anemia. The genes for Fanconi anemia are *FANCC* and *FANCG*, which usually work with the *BRCA2* gene to repair damaged DNA in the cell. When the Fanconi anemia genes are mutated, more breaks in DNA go undetected and allow cancer to develop. Persons with Fanconi anemia often develop leukemia and cancers of the digestive tract, including pancreatic cancer.

Peutz-Jeghers syndrome (PJS). In people with PJS, the risk of digestive tract tumors (esophageal, small bowel, and colorectal) and pancreatic cancer is increased. Polyps in the small intestine and dark spots on the lips and nose are found in persons with PJS. The gene associated with PJS is *STK11/LKB1*. Persons with this syndrome have a 36% risk of developing pancreatic cancer.

Hereditary pancreatitis. This is a rare disease that usually starts at a young age; most cases are diagnosed before age 20. People with hereditary pancreatitis have recurrent episodes of severe inflammation of the pancreas that lead to chronic pancreatitis. The gene associated with this disorder is *PRSS1* (cationic trypsinogen). People with hereditary pancreatitis have a 30% risk of pancreatic cancer. It also has been shown that people with hereditary pancreatitis who smoke may develop earlier onset of pancreatic cancer.

Hereditary nonpolyposis colon cancer (HNPCC; Lynch syndrome). This syndrome is seen in families with colon cancer, generally at a younger age. The specific criteria for HNPCC families who run the risk of pancreatic cancer are that colon cancer occurs in at least three blood relatives, crossing at least two generations, with one of the cancer cases occurring before the age of 50. The genes associated with *HNPCC* are *MSH2* and *MLH1*.

Von Hippel-Lindau syndrome. This is a rare, inherited cancer syndrome associated with the mutated *VHL* gene. People develop renal tumors, adrenal gland tumors, and cysts. The risk of pancreatic cancer is slightly elevated in Von Hippel-Landau syndrome and is usually caused by pancreatic endocrine tumors.

Not everyone who has an inherited change or mutation will develop pancreatic cancer. If you think you are at risk for developing pancreatic cancer, you should discuss this with your healthcare provider or see a genetics counselor, or both.

CHAPTER 2

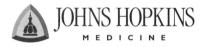

MY TEAM—
MEETING YOUR TREATMENT TEAM

MEMBERS OF A MULTIDISCIPLINARY CARE TEAM

There will be many members of your oncology team to help you with your treatment along this cancer journey. Each member has a specific role and specialty related to pancreatic cancer and its treatment. Here is a list of many of the major members of the team.

Surgical oncologist. A surgeon who specializes in cancer surgery and performs surgery on the pancreas, including the Whipple procedure (pancreaticoduodenectomy); pylorus-preserving Whipple procedure; distal pancreatectomy; central pancreatectomy; laparoscopy for diagnosis, biopsy, and surgery; bowel bypass for palliation; and intraoperative pain blocks (celiac plexus blocks).

Medical oncologist. A doctor who specializes in gastrointestinal cancer (the pancreas is an organ of the gastrointestinal tract) and selects medicines for systemic treatment (treatment that goes to all parts of the body), which includes chemotherapy, targeted therapy, and vaccines. These medicines may be given as part of a clinical trial (research trial). The medicines may be given alone or in combination with various other known or experimental medicines or with radiation therapy. These medicines can be given before or after surgery.

Radiation oncologist. A doctor who specializes in giving radiation to treat cancer. This doctor may have a special interest in gastrointestinal cancer, including pancreatic cancer. Radiation therapy may be given alone or in combination with chemotherapy, either before and/or after surgery. This therapy also can be given at the time of surgery, and it is called intraoperative radiation therapy or intraoperative brachytherapy.

Radiologist. A doctor who reads the X-ray and other imaging studies used to assess what is going on in a person's pancreas as well as other areas in the body. Important imaging studies used to assess a person's pancreas are the CT scan, MRI, MRCP, and PET scan (see Chapter 1).

Endoscopist. A gastroenterologist or surgeon who specializes in performing studies that look at the inside of the gastrointestinal tract by placing a long tube or scope (the endoscope) down your mouth, into the esophagus and the stomach, and then carefully into the first part of the small bowel, called the duodenum. Using special maneuvers and instruments, this doctor can also look into very small areas of the gastrointestinal tract called the common bile duct and main pancreatic duct. These studies help diagnosis by using X-rays and by taking biopsies of any tissues inside these areas of the body. Endoscopes also can be used to place special tubes (stents) to allow the free flow of certain body juices such as bile, pancreatic juice, or stomach contents. If your initial symptoms include jaundice, an endoscopist may be especially important to help relieve your blockage until a decision can be made regarding surgery. Sometimes, this is the first person you may see.

Pathologist. Although you may never meet this doctor, he or she is one of the most important doctors on your team. This doctor looks under the microscope at your biopsy tissue and any tissue taken during surgery to assess the size and type of the cancer, whether cancer has spread to lymph nodes, and whether cancer is at the edges of the tissue taken at surgery. This provides important information that is used to determine your treatment plan and may help predict what will happen in the future.

Anesthesiologist. This doctor puts people to sleep during surgery and also specializes in treating a person's pain problems using medications and certain procedures such as nerve blocks.

Interventional radiologists. Radiologists who have advanced training in the treatment of diseases using radiologic techniques. You may be referred to an interventional radiologist to help place a percutaneous biliary drain (PBD), a tube (stent) in your bile duct to relieve jaundice.

Nurses. A number of nurses will be involved in your care. You will probably meet new ones as you journey through various treatments, which may include surgery, chemotherapy, radiation therapy, clinical trials, vaccines, pain and palliative care, home care, and hospice care. Some of the important functions that nurses perform are providing information; assessing your clinical needs, including pain and other symptoms; providing care for you after surgery; administering chemotherapy drugs; and evaluating your progress during radiation treatment.

Social worker. A person who specializes in patient support, assisting with finding services as well as addressing any psychosocial concerns you may have.

Genetics counselor. An expert in genetics who works with patients and families at risk for hereditary disorders. Genetics counselors work with patients and families to offer information and support, as well as analyze information about genetics issues including risks and inheritance patterns. Patients and families can discuss their genetic testing options with genetics counselors.

Dietician. As nutrition experts, dieticians develop special diets for patients with certain medical issues, including those who cannot consume food normally.

MAKING YOUR INITIAL APPOINTMENT

Making the first appointment may feel overwhelming when you have just learned about your diagnosis of pancreatic cancer. You may not know who or what doctor you should call first. If you were told you were a candidate for surgery, you may want to call a surgeon who specializes in pancreatic surgery.

It is important to choose a surgeon who has experience doing surgery on the pancreas. You have the right to ask questions of the surgeon to decide whether this person is the right doctor for you. It is important to make sure that he or she has board certification and to find out how many pancreatic surgeries he or she does each year. You want a person whose focus is on pancreatic cancer. You also want to find out what the mortality rate (the number of people dying from the operation) is for the surgeon's or institution's patients undergoing pancreatic cancer surgery. Many studies have shown that centers and surgeons that perform this surgery frequently have a significantly lower rate of their patients dying from the Whipple procedure than those who rarely do this operation. If the doctor does not answer your questions or does not know the answers, that may be a signal for you to seek guidance and treatment elsewhere. Be sure the surgeon has performed operations for pancreatic *cancer* and not just pancreas surgery. This is one operation where experience does matter! Unfortunately, less than one-third of people with pancreatic cancer seek out experienced surgeons.

Wherever you make an appointment to be seen, be sure to tell the person helping to arrange your appointment that you have been newly diagnosed with pancreatic cancer. Most places arrange for patient appointments quite promptly. It is not an emergency requiring you to be seen in the next day or two, although you may feel like it is. Your pancreatic cancer has been there for some time. Most estimates suggest that for pancreatic cancer to be seen as a speck on the pancreas on a CT scan it must have already been growing for several years. There are a few exceptions to this rule, but only a few. This means you have time to make good decisions and be sure that you have placed yourself in the best hands. If the place where you are being seen for your pancreatic cancer has a Web site, you may want to look at it and see whether the doctors have their professional information (biographies) posted, in order to learn more about the staff and to determine if there is a particular doctor that you think you may prefer to see.

Some institutions also have established a Pancreas Multidisciplinary Cancer Clinic to help facilitate treatment for patients with pancreatic cancer. You may want to make an appointment directly with the Pancreas Multidisciplinary Cancer Clinic to take advantage of having a complete evaluation by all members of the clinic on one day and to use all of the resources the center has available for patient education, treatment, and research of pancreatic cancer. A patient will:

- Be seen in one location by all services

- Receive a complete assessment

- Have access to many top pancreatic cancer clinicians and research specialists

- Have a recommended plan of treatment by the end of the clinic visit

The goal of the Pancreas Multidisciplinary Cancer Clinic for each patient is:

- To provide a smooth and efficient patient experience

- To improve communication between patients and their healthcare providers

- To improve the quality of life for patients with pancreatic cancer

- To educate patients with pancreatic cancer and their caregivers

- To decrease patient and caregiver anxiety and answer all questions

When you schedule an appointment, be sure to get an address and clear directions for where you need to go and what time you should report there. If you have not been to the place before, allow yourself extra driving time to find it, park, and get to the location where the doctor or doctors will see you. Being late only frustrates you more and your doctor as well. Arriving early gives you time to sit in the waiting area and review your questions one more time to make your visit more productive.

WHAT TO BRING WITH YOU FOR THAT FIRST CONSULTATION

The following information is usually requested to be sent to the doctor's office before your visit, or they may ask you to bring it with you to the first visit:

- Any information about your general health history and a previous physical exam, as well as how you came to see a doctor and what was done to find out that you had a problem with your pancreas. Any recent blood work (laboratory studies), such as electrolyte levels, liver function tests, complete blood count, and levels of any cancer markers (e.g., CA 19-9 and CEA), need to be included.

- A list of the medications you are taking, including vitamins and herbs or anything that you buy over the counter without a prescription.

- A complete list of any previous surgeries, as well as any allergies you may have to medicines or foods.

- Family medical history, especially any pancreas problems or history of pancreatic cancer or any other cancers. If you are not sure about your family history, you may want to call another family member and ask for help in obtaining this information because it is important for your medical summary and may influence some decision making about your treatment recommendations.

- Any X-rays or imaging studies that were done, either the actual X-rays as large films or the images put on a CD, along with the reports; this includes CT scans, MRIs, MRCPs, PET scans, ERCPs, and percutaneous transhepatic cholangiograms (PTCs).

- If you had a pancreas biopsy done or have had previous surgery and had pancreatic tissue taken at the time of surgery, obtain the pathology slides. A biopsy may have been done at the time of an ERCP, EUS, or PTC. If you had a biopsy of another area in your body that was read as cancer from your pancreas that had spread to another part of your body, obtain that biopsy as well. You may have had a biopsy of your liver, lung, lymph node, or a nodule in your abdomen. The pathology slides of the biopsy or biopsies taken may have been requested to be sent in ahead of time, usually by a shipping method that allows a tracking mechanism (such as Federal Express or UPS), with the goal of having the pathologist look at them before you come for your visit and give an opinion about the accuracy of the information provided in the report that came with the biopsy.

You will also need to know in advance whether your insurance company requires you to have preauthorization for having additional tests, such as another CT scan, MRI, or PET scan. There are times when the doctor reviewing the images may find them less than satisfactory. When this occurs, the doctor may want to get additional imaging done while you are there for the visit. You may be told by the facility where the images were originally done that you must bring them back right away. This is not true, because the images are technically your property.

WHO TO BRING WITH YOU TO THE VISIT WITH THE DOCTOR

Bring a trusted family member or friend with you to see the doctor. When people are stressed, they usually only hear and retain 10% of what is said to them. The doctor will be talking and giving you a lot of information. You may be overwhelmed trying to keep it all straight in your mind. The person you bring with you can serve as another set of ears, and can write down what the doctor says. You may want to bring a tape recorder to catch all that is said. Please ask if it is all right to tape anything that is said by any healthcare provider before turning on the recorder. Most healthcare providers are comfortable with the discussion being voice recorded.

QUESTIONS TO ASK DURING YOUR VISIT

Having a list of questions prepared in advance is useful for making the time you have with the doctor as efficient and helpful as possible. Here is a list to help you get started:

1. What type of pancreatic cancer do I have?

2. What stage of disease do you believe I have based on what you know from my clinical examination, X-rays, pathology, and tests done so far?

3. Can my cancer be taken out with surgery, and if so, by what type of pancreatic surgery?

4. Did the pathology team confirm the accuracy of the biopsy results?

5. How soon would my surgery be scheduled?

6. What educational information do you offer to prepare me for surgery and what to expect?

7. Who will be my contact here for questions I may have?

8. Do you have educational materials for other family members, like my children?

9. How many pancreatic cancer surgeries do you perform a year?

10. How long have you been in practice doing pancreatic surgeries?

11. Who else will be involved in my care and when will I meet them?

12. Will I need more therapy (chemotherapy and/or radiation therapy) after surgery? How soon after surgery?

13. How often will I need to see you after my surgery for ongoing evaluation?

14. Are there clinical trials that you recommend for me to consider at this point?

15. Who will be coordinating my care? Do you have a patient navigator?

16. How are future appointments arranged for me and when do these happen?

WILL THERE BE A NEED FOR MORE TESTS?

Another CT scan or MRI may be done at the facility where you are being seen because the quality of all scans, as well as the expertise of the radiologist reading the scans, is not equal. Places with a high number of patients being seen and treated for pancreatic cancer have been shown to have higher rates of accuracy in reading scans and pathology slides, and a better long-term survival rate. Currently, a 64-slice multidetector row spiral (or helical) CT scan using a special pancreas protocol with a three-dimensional reconstruction is considered state of the art for imaging the pancreas and related blood vessels, organs, and nearby tissues. Do not be surprised if further tests are needed, because you want the doctors to be thorough. The idea of needing more tests can be stressful, but it is important to have the best information before proceeding on any treatment, including surgery.

All this information provides more detail about the pancreas and where the cancer is located. This allows the doctor to decide whether you should undergo surgery to remove the cancer. If surgery is not an option, then further evaluation for treatment will be done by the medical oncologist and radiation oncologist. Sometimes, a surgeon may feel that a cancer cannot be removed because it's very close to or involved with major blood vessels, such as the superior mesenteric vein. In this case, getting a second opinion is a good idea to make sure that another surgeon who may be more experienced in pancreatic cancer surgery agrees.

A biopsy of the pancreas or another area in the body may need to be done to obtain tumor tissue to see the type of actual cancer cells. This is needed before any chemotherapy, radiation therapy, or clinical trial can start to best know how to treat your cancer. You usually do not need to know the actual cancer cell type (see pages 4–5) before having surgery because you will get that information when the tumor is removed at surgery. In some cases, a diagnosis of pancreatic cancer cannot be made despite many attempts at obtaining a biopsy, and a surgeon will then operate to remove the pancreatic mass if the mass in your pancreas looks worrisome.

If your tumor can be removed by surgery, additional blood work and tests related to preparing for surgery may be needed. The preoperative tests may include chest X-ray, electrocardiogram (EKG), type and crossmatch for blood, and urinalysis. These are not tests specifically related to a diagnosis of cancer but are done routinely for anyone having an operation. Consultations for specific functions of the body, such as heart, lung, and kidney, may also be requested to make sure these organs are working adequately before you have surgery.

HOW BEST TO CONTACT TEAM MEMBERS

Request business cards from each healthcare provider you see and ask what their office procedure is for responding to questions or concerns you may have. Usually there is one contact person on whom you can rely to address your questions. Find out also if you can communicate with any of the team by email. If and when the need arises to contact the team with questions, be concise and think all your thoughts through. It is better to ask three questions at once rather then one question three different times in a row.

NAVIGATING APPOINTMENTS

Some cancer centers may have patient navigators. A patient navigator may have different roles in different facilities, such as assisting with scheduling appointments, getting test results back, helping to get surgery scheduled, arranging for you to see a medical and/or radiation oncologist before or after surgery, and in general, being available for support as well as to address other clinical and psychosocial needs that may arise. In some cases your point person may be a nurse in the doctor's office, the office manager in the doctor's office, or the doctor assigned for your chemotherapy or radiation therapy. In other cases the contact person may be called a case manager, who usually functions just like a navigator. The title isn't important, but having the ability to call someone who can help you with your questions and appointment details is.

FINANCIAL IMPLICATIONS OF TREATMENT/ INSURANCE CLEARANCE

You did not plan on getting diagnosed with pancreatic cancer. There is no convenient time to get this disease. The disease alone can raise havoc in your life. If you are working outside the home, you will be taking time off for any treatments. It is useful to find out about your health insurance coverage and your workplace's policy about time off from work ahead of time. Finding out about how much sick leave you have, along with short-term disability coverage, copayment information, prescription coverage, and other medical expense issues, is helpful for planning your future needs.

Your insurance company may require you to obtain referrals in order to see certain specialists, get tests done, or have surgery authorized, as well as other treatments and medications. If you need help with these things, a social worker may assist you. Please ask for the help of a social worker. A financial assistant also may be available to help with these issues. Some treatments that are recommended may be related to clinical trials; some of these may be covered by your insurance, and others may not. If you participate in a clinical trial, a research nurse will assist you with insurance information.

Financial issues are always a concern, and the availability of financial support is not always well advertised. You will need to ask to see whether there is anything in your state or area for financial support. Be proactive in asking to meet with a social worker to discuss what support services may be available to you.

You can find information about pancreatic cancer and the Pancreas Multidisciplinary Cancer Clinic at Johns Hopkins Hospital at http://www.path.jhu.edu/pancreas/.

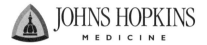

CHAPTER 3

TAKING ACTION—
COMPREHENSIVE TREATMENT
CONSIDERATIONS

This chapter describes the various types of treatment available for adenocarcinomas of the pancreas and the decision making involved in determining whether you need that treatment or not. As mentioned previously, endocrine tumors of the pancreas will not be discussed here. However, the surgical resection techniques for endocrine cancers of the pancreas are similar to those described here (although the prognosis for such cancers may be better). Pancreatic cancer treatment can include surgery, chemotherapy, targeted therapy, radiation therapy, vaccine therapy, pain management, palliative therapies, and clinical trials. The first step in choosing your therapy is finding the right team of physicians. You should seek treatment for your cancer in centers that treat a large number of patients with pancreatic cancer. Many studies have shown that patients do better when they are treated at these so-called high-volume centers.

SURGICAL TREATMENT

Surgery remains the primary treatment to cure patients of pancreatic cancer. Surgery involves removal of the cancer along with surrounding lymph nodes. Surgery is usually an option for early stages (Stage 0, I, or II) of pancreatic cancer when the cancer has not spread to other distant organs (such as the liver or lungs, called metastasis) and the cancer does not involve major blood vessels such as the arteries. If major veins are involved, it is sometimes still possible to perform surgery by doing a vein resection.

Once you meet your surgeon, he or she will need to review the images from a good-quality multidetector CT scan (as discussed in Chapter 1) to determine whether the tumor can be removed. If the tumor can be removed, it is called resectable. About 15% to 20% of patients with pancreatic cancers have tumors that are resectable. For the rest of patients, surgery may still be required to relieve blockages of the bile duct or stomach, referred to as a palliative bypass procedure. The type of surgery selected to remove the pancreatic cancer depends on the location of the tumor within the pancreas. These surgical procedures include the Whipple procedure, distal pancreatectomy, total pancreatectomy, and palliative bypass.

WHIPPLE PROCEDURE

The Whipple procedure, or pancreaticoduodenectomy, is the most common surgery performed for pancreatic cancer. It is done for surgical treatment of a cancer found in the head or uncinate process of the pancreas. About 75% of pancreatic cancers are found in this location. See Figure 2 for a detailed anatomy of the pancreas.

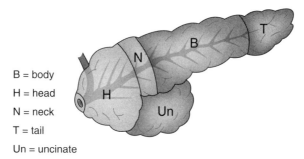

B = body
H = head
N = neck
T = tail
Un = uncinate

Figure 2 The pancreas.

Adapted from artwork by Jennifer Parsons Brumbaugh from http://pathology.jhu.edu/pancreas.

During the Whipple operation, the surgeon removes the cancer within the pancreas along with its surrounding lymph nodes. Currently, many centers perform the pylorus-preserving Whipple procedure (see Figure 3), in which the surgeon removes the following:

- Head of the pancreas

- Lymph nodes draining that area of the pancreas

- Part of the bile duct (a tube that drains bile from the liver into the small bowel)

- Gallbladder

- Most of the duodenum (which is the first part of the small bowel)

The stomach is saved, along with the first portion of the duodenum.

Some surgeons may perform a classic Whipple; in this case, the surgery involves the above procedures as well as removal of the entire duodenum, along with a small portion of the stomach. Regardless of the type of Whipple

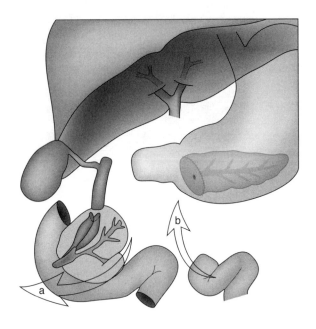

Figure 3 a) Duodenum, head of pancreas, bile duct, and gallbladder removed. b) Jejunum raised.

Adapted from artwork by Jennifer Parsons Brumbaugh from http://pathology. jhu.edu/pancreas.

procedure performed, the goal is to remove the entire tumor. After the tumor is removed, the surgeon then has to reconnect the remaining pancreas, the remaining bile duct, and the stomach (in a classic Whipple) or the remaining part of the duodenum (in a pylorus-preserving Whipple) to the small intestine (see Figure 4). This allows the digestive enzymes produced in the pancreas, bile, and stomach contents to flow into the small intestines for normal digestion.

The Whipple operation usually takes 5 to 8 hours. Most patients will stay in the hospital for 7 to 10 days. You may spend 1 or 2 nights in an intensive care unit (ICU). You may have several devices attached to you to monitor your blood

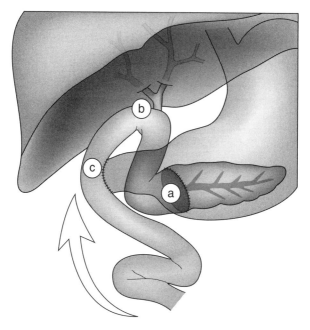

Figure 4   Jejunum reattached to a) Pancreas, b) Hepatic duct, c) Duodenum.

Adapted from artwork by Jennifer Parsons Brumbaugh from http://pathology. jhu.edu/pancreas.

pressure, heart rate, and urine. You may also have abdominal drains placed around the area of your surgery. A tube called a nasogastric (NG) tube is usually placed in your nose at the time of surgery. The nurses will also check your blood sugar levels regularly since the pancreas produces insulin, which helps adjust your blood sugar. Most people will not become diabetic from this surgery if they did not have diabetes before surgery. If you already have diabetes, your medications may need to be adjusted after surgery.

The pathology report will usually be available within a week after your surgery. It will help determine the stage of your cancer. The surgeon may perform a "frozen section" on a piece of tumor taken in the operating room to give a pre-liminary idea of whether this is a cancer or a benign tumor.

As mentioned earlier, high-volume centers can now per-form this operation safely with a mortality of 1% to 2%, whereas low-volume centers have a surgical mortality rate four times that. One of the most common complications that are seen after a Whipple procedure is delayed gastric emptying (DGE), in which the stomach does not empty properly. This is seen in about one in every six patients having the procedure. This condition will typically resolve within 7 to 10 days, and you may need to have an NG tube placed in your nose to empty stomach secretions.

Another complication that may be seen in about 1 in 10 patients is a pancreatic leak, in which there is leakage of pancreatic juice from the connection of the pancreas to the small intestine. This can result in an abdominal infection and may require antibiotics and placement of drains by an interventional radiologist to remove the pancreatic secre-tions. You might not be able to eat anything by mouth for a short time while the pancreatic connection heals. You will then be fed by an IV with total parenteral nutrition, also called TPN, or by a feeding tube during that interim.

Patients who have undergone the Whipple procedure take a while to recover, ranging from a few weeks to months. You may be asked to take pancreatic enzymes to help with digestion. These are pills (usually one or two) taken with each meal to allow you to digest the fat from your meal. Taking pancreatic enzymes may be necessary for a few months to a lifetime. The amount can be adjusted, so if you know you are going out to a restaurant and having a big meal, you may want to take extra enzyme pills.

DISTAL PANCREATECTOMY

A distal pancreatectomy is performed when the cancer is located in the body or tail of the pancreas. The surgeon will remove the body and tail of the pancreas, and often the spleen as well. The goal is to remove the cancer with negative margins and remove local lymph nodes. The cut end of the pancreas is closed with sutures or staples. The most common complication with a distal pancreatectomy is a pancreatic leak from the cut end of the pancreas, which is treated as mentioned earlier. If your spleen was removed, you will receive several vaccines before you leave the hospital to help you fight certain type of infections such as pneumonia. Patients can also have the vaccines given to them a couple of weeks before surgery.

LAPAROSCOPIC SURGERY

In some patients, surgery to remove the pancreatic cancer can be performed laparoscopically. This type of procedure is currently best suited for small cancers in the tail of the pancreas. In addition, a laparoscopic procedure is often used for very large cancers in the tail of the pancreas to look for spread of the cancer (or metastasis) to other organs. If such metastases are encountered, then the patient can be spared a larger incision because major surgery is not indicated and the patient would benefit more from systemic chemotherapy. Some of the benefits of a laparoscopic procedure are that it allows for a smaller incision and may improve recovery because there is less pain after the surgery. However, the pancreas is a difficult organ to work with and prone to bleeding. Patients are encouraged to seek out a pancreatic surgeon who is also experienced in laparoscopic surgery.

TOTAL PANCREATECTOMY

A total pancreatectomy is done to remove the entire pancreas because of a cancer in the head or uncinate process of the pancreas or throughout the pancreas. This procedure is similar to a Whipple procedure in that parts of the bile duct and the gallbladder and the majority of the duodenum are removed (or the entire duodenum and part of the stomach, as in a classic Whipple), but now the entire pancreas is removed. The surgeon still has to reconnect the remaining bile duct and the stomach (as in a classic Whipple) or the remaining part of the duodenum (as in a pylorus-preserving Whipple) to the small intestine. The spleen is usually removed as well.

You will become diabetic after this procedure because the entire pancreas is gone, and you will need to take insulin for the rest of your life. You should be seen by a diabetic educator and have follow-up with an endocrinologist for your diabetes management. You will also need to take pancreatic enzymes for the rest of your life to help in the digestion of fatty foods. An insulin pump may be placed to help manage your blood sugar levels after you have recovered fully from the total pancreatectomy.

NEOADJUVANT THERAPY

Sometimes, the pancreatic cancer is considered to be "borderline" resectable when it has spread to nearby lymph nodes or it is near major blood vessels, such as when the cancer surrounds more than half the circumference of the superior mesenteric vein (Stages IIB and III). In such cases, your surgeon may elect to give you neoadjuvant (before surgery) treatment to help shrink the cancer and allow it to be removed. Neoadjuvant treatment usually includes a combination of radiation therapy and chemotherapy. Delivery of neoadjuvant therapy requires a multidisciplinary team that works together closely with the surgeon to monitor the response of the cancer to therapy.

ADJUVANT THERAPY

Adjuvant therapy is additional treatment after surgical removal of the pancreatic cancer and generally includes treatment in the form of chemotherapy and radiation therapy. In addition, immunotherapy and other targeted biologic therapies may be selectively used. Most patients with pancreatic cancer will be recommended to undergo adjuvant therapy once they have recovered from surgery, a process that usually takes at least 6 weeks. The type and length of time of adjuvant treatment will depend on the stage of the disease, the age of the patient, and the general health of the patient. Other prognostic factors will be determined by the pathologist after examining the cancer obtained from surgery.

PALLIATIVE PROCEDURES

Surgical Bypass

Sometimes pancreatic cancer has already spread to other organs (metastasized), or the cancer is locally advanced and cannot be safely removed. In these cases, surgery to alleviate symptoms of jaundice or nausea and vomiting is needed. A biliary bypass may be performed. The surgery bypasses the area where the bile duct is blocked by connecting a part of the bile duct to an area of the small intestine so the bile can drain into the intestine and help with normal digestion.

In some patients, the cancer may cause blockage of the duodenum or the stomach, called gastric outlet obstruction, which causes profound nausea and vomiting because any food or liquids taken cannot pass out of the stomach into the intestine. A gastric bypass connects the unaffected stomach to part of the small intestine to relieve the blockage. If the cancer blocks both the bile duct and the stomach outlet, a palliative double bypass is performed.

Patients who suffer from these blockages may have abdominal and back pain from the cancer growing into the nerves in this area. If one or both bypasses are performed, a special pain management procedure, called a celiac block, can be performed during surgery to help with abdominal and back pain. In this procedure, the surgeon injects alcohol into the major nerve around the pancreas, called the celiac nerve. This type of block can provide substantial relief from pain and can last several months. The celiac block can be repeated, as needed, in the future. The same procedure can be done by an anesthesia pain specialist. The procedure can be done on an outpatient basis without requiring formal surgery.

Stents

Blockage of the bile duct or the stomach can be relieved without surgery by placing stents to bypass the blockage. Stents can be placed across the blockage in the bile duct or duodenum to relieve the obstruction. These stents are made of plastic or metal. Generally, plastic stents will only stay patent (open) for a short time and can be removed and a new stent placed, whereas metal stents may last longer but cannot be removed. The stent can cause an infection, because it is a foreign object in the body and can collect debris inside it or be placed improperly in the bile duct. In such cases, patients may have fevers and chills and develop jaundice (referred to as cholangitis) if the stent was placed in the bile duct. If you suspect a stent infection, you need to contact your doctor immediately, since these infections can be serious.

CHEMOTHERAPY

Chemotherapy drugs are given to eradicate or kill cancer cells. They are systemic therapies—that is, they get into the bloodstream and kill all rapidly dividing cells such as cancer cells, but they can also affect other dividing, healthy cells. The side effects of chemotherapy are related to the damage they cause to normal healthy cells. Medications are available to help treat most of the common side effects of chemotherapy.

Chemotherapy is an important component of treatment for all stages of pancreatic cancer. Chemotherapy is given by itself after surgery to improve survival, and is also often combined with radiation and is referred to as adjuvant therapy. In patients for whom surgery is not feasible, chemotherapy is used alone or in combination with other treatments such as targeted therapy, radiation therapy, and immunotherapy.

Chemotherapy can be given intravenously (the drug is placed into a vein to be delivered into the bloodstream) or orally (by mouth). Most patients receive chemotherapy as an outpatient in either a hospital clinic or a doctor's office. Most chemotherapy regimens are given every few weeks, and the length needed for each type of drug will vary. Medical oncologists are physicians who specialize in treating patients with chemotherapy for cancer.

The standard chemotherapy at present is a drug called Gemzar (gemcitabine). Gemzar is administered by the IV route and was approved in 1996 as standard treatment for pancreatic cancer. It is indicated as a first-line treatment for patients with locally advanced (stage II or III) cancer who are not candidates for surgery and for patients with metastatic (stage IV) cancer.

Before the use of Gemzar, most patients were treated with 5-fluorouracil (5-FU). In a landmark study published in the *Journal of the American Medical Association*, it was shown that the addition of Gemzar to adjuvant fluorouracil-based chemoradiation was associated with a survival benefit for patients with resected pancreatic cancer of about 3.5 months, compared with patients who were treated with 5-fluorouracil in addition to chemoradiation. Currently, there are many promising studies trying to improve upon the results obtained from the single-agent Gemzar alone. Most of these combinations will be available in the context of a clinical trial.

Talk with your medical oncologist about what steps can be taken to reduce possible side effects from chemotherapy. Not everyone experiences side effects. Medications are available to prevent or dramatically reduce nausea. Exercise has been proven to help reduce the side effect of fatigue. (See Chapter 4 for more information on side effects.) Generally, most patients feel well the day of the treatment. If side effects are going to occur, they most commonly happen the night chemotherapy is given or the next day.

During your chemotherapy treatment, your blood will be taken at designated intervals to make sure that your red blood cells and white blood cells are staying within normal limits. If they are low, which is a common side effect, the doctor might decide to give you special medicines to boost your blood counts back to a normal range. Also, be careful of being around people who have a cold or flu, because your immune system is being strained when you are undergoing chemotherapy treatment. Finally, remember that there is a beginning and an end to taking chemotherapy. We can deal with anything when we know it is only for a designated period of time.

RADIATION THERAPY

Radiation therapy is provided by specialized doctors called radiation oncologists. Radiation oncologists use high-energy X-rays to treat the area of the cancer along with a small area of normal surrounding tissue. Radiation therapy is a way to treat the cancer directly, also called local treatment. Radiation therapy is used to prevent the cancer from coming back (local recurrence) in patients whose cancer was removed. In patients whose pancreatic cancer has been removed, radiation therapy is given as adjuvant therapy, usually with low-dose chemotherapy, termed chemoradiation. It is important to understand that the dose of chemotherapy that is given in chemoradiation acts as a radiosensitizer; that is, the chemotherapy dose is really meant to help the radiation be more effective, and you will likely need additional chemotherapy in larger doses after chemoradiation is over.

The chemotherapy drugs that are used as radiation sensitizers include 5-fluorouracil and Gemzar. In patients whose cancer is locally advanced and there is concern that surgery may not be feasible, radiation is given along with chemotherapy as a neoadjuvant treatment to help shrink the cancer and possibly allow the cancer to be surgically removed. Finally, radiation therapy may also be used in patients with metastatic disease for palliation to relieve pain.

Radiation therapy is generally given 5 days a week for several weeks, ranging from 2 to 6 weeks. The treatment is given on an outpatient basis in a clinic. Before radiation begins, you will have some special measurements done, called simulation, to ensure that the radiation beams are always lined up the same way to radiate the same area consistently and precisely. A few tiny tattoo marks (little blue dots) will be made on your abdomen as part of the preparation process. These dots are usually permanent.

Radiation doesn't hurt. It feels similar to getting a chest X-ray, which means you feel nothing at all. However, radiation is cumulative (builds up over time); that's why you may start getting fatigued toward the last few weeks of treatment. Exercising regularly, such as power walking, has been proven to reduce this specific side effect. There have been vast improvements in radiation therapy over the last decade. Special technology is used so that only the tissues that need to be radiated are treated.

The use of radiation therapy in the treatment of pancreatic cancer is debated in the medical literature, since clinical trials in the United States and in Europe have shown variable benefits from radiation therapy. Generally, in the United States most patients are given radiation therapy, whereas it's rarely used in Europe. Finally, delivery of radiation therapy requires skill in ensuring that normal tissues are not exposed to X-rays and avoiding any toxicity of the therapy. This is especially important for pancreatic cancer patients since the pancreas is a small organ that is surrounded by many vital structures. Patients are encouraged to find centers that have experience in treating patients with pancreatic cancer.

IMMUNOTHERAPY

Immunotherapy refers to therapies that stimulate the body's own immune system to help fight cancer. All cancers arise from our normal cells due to the accumulation of defects in their genes. Immunotherapy, thus, has a lot of potential in the treatment of cancers. The goals of immunotherapy are to enhance the body's immune response to stop or slow down tumor growth and to make tumors more amenable to responding to therapy. At present, immunotherapy is delivered in the form of vaccines for pancreatic cancer and has shown some limited benefit.

The pancreatic cancer vaccine, unlike vaccines for childhood infections, is a vaccine used to treat existing disease. Pancreatic cancer must already have been diagnosed for this vaccine to work. The vaccination causes an immune response that targets any pancreatic cancer cells.

TARGETED BIOLOGICAL THERAPY

In recent years, clinical trials have been completed that evaluated the effect of targeted biological therapy either instead of chemotherapy or in combination with chemotherapy agents. Targeted biological therapies are aimed at characteristics unique to cancer cells, allowing the therapy to attack cancer cells more directly and effectively while simultaneously avoiding the toxicity of chemotherapy to normal cells.

One of the targeted biological therapies used for the treatment of advanced pancreatic cancer is Tarceva (erlotinib) used in combination with Gemzar. Tarceva is a small molecule that is designed to target the human epidermal growth factor type 1/epidermal growth factor receptor (HER1/EGFR). HER1, also known as EGFR, is a component of the HER signaling pathway, which plays a critical role in the formation and growth of some pancreatic cancers. A large clinical trial showed that patients with advanced pancreatic cancer who were treated with Tarceva in addition to Gemzar had modest improvement in 1-year survival rates compared with patients treated with Gemzar alone. Most other targeted biological therapies are in clinical trials.

CLINICAL TRIALS

New and innovative treatments are developed and implemented by performing clinical trials. Without clinical trials we could not improve the treatment of pancreatic cancer, nor could we develop ways to prevent it in the future. Clinical trials are the backbone of science today. Your doctors may at any given time during your treatment discuss with you opportunities to participate in a clinical trial. Be open-minded! Hear what is being offered as part of a study. Let's begin, though, by educating you about what we mean by the term "clinical trials."

There are many different kinds of clinical trials. They range from studies focusing on ways to prevent pancreatic cancer to studies on how to detect, diagnose, and treat it. Most clinical trials are carried out in phases. Each phase is designed to learn different information and build on the information previously discovered. Patients may be eligible for studies in different phases depending on their stage of disease, anticipated therapies, and the treatment they have already had. Patients are monitored at specific intervals while participating in studies.

Phase I studies are used to find the best way to do a new treatment and how much of it can be given safely (optimum dose). In such studies only a small number of patients are asked to participate. Phase I studies are offered to patients whose cancer cannot be helped by other known treatment modalities. These patients usually have metastatic pancreatic cancer and have exhausted other treatment options. Some patients receive benefit from participation in this kind of study, but most experience no benefit in fighting their cancer. However, all are paving the way for the next generation of patients, which is important. Once the optimum dose is chosen, the drug is studied for its ability to shrink tumors in phase II trials.

Phase II studies are designed to find out whether the treatment actually kills cancer cells in patients. A slightly larger number of patients are selected for this type of trial, usually between 20 and 50. Patients whose pancreatic cancer no longer responds to other known treatments may be offered participation in this type of trial. Tumor shrinkage is measured, and patients are closely observed to measure the effects the treatment is having on their disease. If at least a predefined percentage (usually 15% to 20%) of patients in this type of study responds to treatment, the treatment is considered to be successful. Side effects are also closely monitored and carefully recorded and addressed.

Phase III studies usually compare standard treatments already in use with treatments that appeared to be good in phase II trials. This phase requires large numbers of patients to participate (hundreds to thousands). Patients are usually randomized into groups for the treatment regimen they will be receiving. These studies are seeking the benefits of longer survival, fewer side effects, and fewer cases of cancer recurrence. This is the most common type of clinical trial you may hear about and be offered an opportunity to participate in.

Below are a list of questions that you should consider asking to help guide you in decision making and fact finding about clinical trials:

What is the purpose of the study?

How many people will be included in the study?

What does the study involve? What kind of tests and treatment will I have?

How are treatments given and what side effects might I expect?

What are the risks and benefits of each protocol?

What alternatives do I have to participating in the study?

How long will the study last?

What type of long-term follow-up care is provided for those who participate?

Will I incur any costs? Will my insurance company pay for part of this?

When will the results be known?

Every successful cancer treatment being used today started as a clinical trial. Those patients who participated in these studies were the first to benefit. Participation can therefore potentially benefit you, but perhaps equally important (and to others more important) may be the opportunity to contribute in a major way for the next generation of patients having to deal with pancreatic cancer.

Clinical trials are taking place in many parts of the country. Information about ongoing clinical trials is available from the NCI Web site. Choosing the most appropriate clinical trial is a decision that ideally involves you, your family, and your healthcare team.

CHAPTER 4

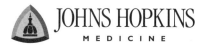

BE PREPARED—THE SIDE EFFECTS OF TREATMENT

N ow that you have heard your diagnosis and it's starting to sink in, you must be filled with questions about what happens next, what to expect, and what your life is going to be like. These questions are normal and will be addressed in this chapter. Although your questions can be addressed in general, be aware that *every* patient handles treatment—whether it is surgery, chemotherapy, or radiation—in a different manner. Different patients can receive the same chemotherapy medication and react in many different ways. Friends and family may say things like "When so-and-so had chemotherapy, this is what happened to him or her." Remember, *you* are an individual with your own journey, and your body will react in an individual way. There are *many* different chemotherapy medications, each with its own side effects. You may not be receiving the same medication that others have received or in the same doses and, therefore, may not have the same side effects. You need to realize that you are different.

Perhaps you have heard of or seen someone taking chemotherapy many years ago who experienced a lot of nausea and vomiting, and you are worried that this is going to happen to you as well. Things have changed over the years, however, and there are now many medications that can be given to prevent nausea and vomiting. You can continue to live your life while receiving chemotherapy.

Nausea and vomiting *can* be side effects of the medication you are receiving. If this is the case, you will be given medication to take at home for these side effects. Sometimes, more than one medication is given so you can have relief. If you experience nausea, *do not wait* to take the medication, because nausea from chemotherapy only increases. It does not come in waves, like other nausea you may have had before, and the medications will take longer to kick in and bring relief. Make sure you are taking the medication as directed even if you don't like to take a lot of medicine. It is important to feel well and eat properly when on chemotherapy, which you cannot do when you are feeling nauseated or are vomiting. You can stop taking these medications when you have finished chemotherapy and nausea is no longer an issue.

If you are taking the medication properly and are still nauseated or vomiting, you need to call your nurse or doctor and report this to see whether there is anything else that can be done. If you are experiencing nausea, here are some suggestions:

• Make sure you do not allow too much time to elapse before eating. Having an empty stomach may cause nausea by itself, so eat something, even if it is something small such as saltine crackers, broth, or Jell-O.

- Eat small amounts of food more frequently throughout the day.

- Drink liquids before or after eating solid food.

- Eat bland foods such as crackers, chicken noodle soup, plain rice, and scrambled eggs.

- Avoid fatty, greasy foods because they are harder to digest.

Remember, *not every patient receiving chemotherapy has nausea*. This is just a potential side effect.

One question that many patients ask is "Am I going to lose my hair?" Not every chemotherapy medication makes you lose your hair. Your doctor or nurse will be able to answer this question when it is decided exactly what medication you will be receiving. If you are not going to lose your hair, it will get thinner and more brittle the longer you receive chemotherapy. Ask your doctor or nurse if you are thinking about coloring or treating your hair, because these chemicals can be hard on your hair follicles while you are taking chemotherapy. If you are going to lose your hair, wigs can be made that look very real and fit your face. Check with your insurance company, because some insurance companies will pay for wigs needed as a result of hair loss during chemotherapy; you will need a prescription from your doctor, however.

One of the main complaints from patients on chemotherapy, regardless of their diagnosis, is fatigue. This happens for a number of reasons. First, your body always wants to be balanced and will be working hard to achieve that balance even while you are on treatment. Chemotherapy cannot tell the difference between cancer cells and "good" cells in your body such as white blood cells, red blood cells, and platelets. Chemotherapy kills fast-growing cells, which include the "good" cells *and* cancer cells. Your body will want to make more "good" cells to keep in balance and will work hard to make these in your bone marrow. The other reason you may be tired is because when you have low numbers of red blood cells, which can happen while on chemotherapy, you become anemic. Red blood cells give us energy, carry oxygen to all the cells in our body, and make us feel better. When the red blood cell count is low, you can feel fatigued. Sometimes you may need a medication to boost your red blood cell production, and at other times you may need a blood transfusion. Your doctor or nurse will talk about this with you if this situation occurs.

Listen to your body and take rest periods when you are feeling tired. If you are used to running around all day, you may have to stop and rest at times throughout the day. If you are at the mall, you may need to sit and rest for some time before continuing shopping. You can work while receiving chemotherapy, but know that when you get home you will be more tired than usual. Some companies are very good about working with you while you are on treatment and will take your fatigue into consideration.

If you are in a chair or bed all the time, something is wrong, and you need to call your doctor or nurse. You should be able to do your activities, but should plan more time for rest if you need it. Do not push yourself to the point of exhaustion; it takes a lot longer to recover from this extreme fatigue. You are probably asking "How will I know when to rest?" Listen to your body—it's a wonderful machine and will tell you when to rest.

Perhaps you had already lost some weight before you were diagnosed. This is not uncommon prior to diagnosis. It is important for you to try to maintain (or gain) weight while you are receiving chemotherapy. If you are having loose stools about 30 to 45 minutes after eating or are having oily, floating stools, or if you are experiencing abdominal pain with bloating after you eat, let your doctor or nurse know. Sometimes people with pancreatic cancer need enzymes in the form of medication to help digest their food. The pancreas is very important in releasing enzymes when you eat to aid in the digestion and absorption of food. When you have a cancer in the pancreas, it can block the normal production of these enzymes. Your doctor or nurse will instruct you on how to take this medication should you need it.

Try to eat healthy foods, such as fruits, vegetables, grains, dairy products, and protein. Protein is essential in repairing cells, and those "good" cells will need repairing. If you need to gain weight, here are some suggestions:

- Eat smaller meals more frequently.

- Snack on nuts, peanut butter, and cheese. These add calories but will not fill you up.

- Use butter on your food.

- Eat cream soups instead of plain soups because they add more calories.

- Use whole milk instead of fat-free milk.

- Use Boost, Ensure, or Carnation Instant Breakfast (with whole milk) and add ice cream for a shake. This should be taken along with your meals. If you are a diabetic, you could try sugar-free versions, such as Glucerna.

If you are having trouble digesting the fatty foods just listed, let your doctor or nurse know because you may need to take pancreatic enzymes to help digest these foods.

Many patients experience an increase in gas and bloating. This is not from the chemotherapy but because of issues with digestion related to pancreatic cancer. Watch out for gas-producing foods such as onions, cabbage, broccoli, beans, and carbonated drinks. Check with your doctor or nurse to see if you can use Gas-X or Beano to help ease this problem. If you are not having these problems, feel free to enjoy those foods.

You might have heard the term "chemo brain" already, and if you haven't yet, you probably will during your treatment. Some patients who are receiving chemotherapy have, at times, trouble remembering simple things such as names, phone numbers, what they were looking for, and so on. Don't worry; this will usually get better when your chemotherapy is finished. It is not clear why this occurs, but there is beginning to be more written about this topic. Some patients find it helpful to write notes to remind them of things, keep calendars, and get family members or friends to help with reminders. If you experience more than simple forgetfulness or are experiencing any other symptoms, you need to let your doctor or nurse know right away.

Some chemotherapy medications can cause a side effect called neuropathy, which is a numbness and tingling in your hands and feet, similar to when your hand or foot falls asleep. It usually starts in your fingertips and toes and can move up these extremities. Some of the sensation will return when chemotherapy is completed, but it may not go away completely. Let your doctor or nurse know if you are starting to experience this feeling. Treatment is usually not stopped because of this side effect unless it is becoming a problem. If you are having trouble buttoning things or writing, you need to let your doctor or nurse know.

A minor, irritating, side effect of chemotherapy can be a metallic taste in your mouth. Some patients say this is what causes their nausea. Anything with lemon will help cut the metallic taste. Try lemon drops, lemon in water, lemon-flavored Italian ices, and marinating foods (such as chicken) in lemon. Patients say this really helps their taste buds. Also try using plastic silverware instead of metal silverware. Do not use mouthwash that contains alcohol because this dries your mouth and can make it more prone to mouth sores. Use mouthwash without alcohol, such as Biotene or Crest.

Some of you may be saying, "Well, I'm getting radiation along with my chemotherapy—what is that going to be like?" You will have a separate team of doctors and nurses that only work with the radiation part of your treatment, and you will have a chemotherapy doctor and nurse as well. These two teams work together to ensure your treatment goes smoothly. The amount of radiation treatment you will receive will depend on the treatment plan that is best for you. The first half of radiation treatment is fairly easy for most patients; it is the last half that may cause some problems. During the last half of the treatment, you may experience more fatigue and nausea. Again, your doctor and nurse can adjust your medications and suggest other things to make this time easier for you. It is important for you to be totally honest about how you are feeling.

At times, during your treatment, your chemotherapy may have to be postponed (held) if your white blood cell or platelet counts are low. Do not panic; this is not dangerous. Your doctor has to make sure your body will be able to tolerate the treatment, and if these numbers are too low, it is telling us that your body is not able to take the chemotherapy at the moment. There may be a time when your chemotherapy dose has to be reduced as well because your "good cells" continue to be low on a regular basis. Again, do not panic; it is better to get a dose reduction and get your chemotherapy on time than to have a situation in which the chemotherapy has to be held.

You are now ready to begin your treatment. If this chapter has produced more questions, write them down and bring them with you to your first treatment so they can be answered. No question is too small, and knowledge gives you power. This is your journey, but you are not alone. You will have lots of support from your chemotherapy and/or radiation therapy team who will guide you through this experience.

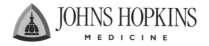

CHAPTER 5

JOHNS HOPKINS
MEDICINE

STRAIGHT TALK—
COMMUNICATION WITH FAMILY,
FRIENDS, AND COWORKERS
BY ELLA-MAE SHUPE, RN

You are probably still overwhelmed and in shock over your diagnosis. Every patient feels this way, and many people say, "But I'm not sick—how can I have cancer?" Pancreatic cancer is one of those "silent" cancers in which the symptoms are vague and could be just normal, everyday things that happen to people, such as bloating, weight loss, loose stools, or mild abdominal pain. Some people do not feel anything until they become jaundiced (have yellow skin color), or constant abdominal pain, at which time the cancer is often discovered.

At this point, you are still trying to understand this news yourself and tell those you love about your diagnosis. If you have children, this can be particularly hard because, as a parent, you want to always protect your children from pain. As you tell your family, expect them to feel the same shock, disappointment, and fear that you are facing. As family members, they may feel helpless because there is not much they can do at this point to make you feel better, and they may feel like they just want to "fix it" for you. It can be hard on family to see you sad, crying, and coping with this, but it is important for you to go through these emotions as well.

Expect to have good days where you feel like you are coping well with the situation and bad days where you are not dealing well with it at all—*this is normal*. This pattern may continue throughout your treatment: good days and bad days. If you are having a hard time dealing with this, feel sad and depressed most days, are in bed most of the day, and aren't eating and sleeping well, you probably need some guidance in coping. You can ask your nurse or doctor to assist you with finding someone, or you can seek outside counseling from someone you know and trust. Some patients may need medications to help them through this time; again, *this is okay!* It does not mean you can't handle it or are weak; it will just help restore you to a place where life is not so overwhelming. Everyone copes with crises in a different manner. How you cope with it is *your* way. People bring all of their experiences with them when they deal with stress, and cancer can be stressful.

When you talk to your children, make the communication age-specific. Tell them the truth (if you feel you can and this is best for your family) but do not scare them. Explain your treatment plan and how you are going to fight the cancer at this time. Some younger children (ages 4 to 7, but most commonly 3- to 5-year-olds) have fantasy thoughts (magical thinking) and may think they caused the illness. Assure your children that they had nothing to do with this diagnosis. It sounds silly, but a child's brain works in different ways. Tell the child it is okay to ask you questions or tell you thoughts he or she may be having. There are resources available to help you with this type of communication, so feel free to ask your nurse or doctor to get you in contact with those resources.

If you are telling teenagers, remember that in their minds the world is all about them. They will be anxious and worry about the impact of your disease and treatment on their world and their activities. They also may worry about their safe world not feeling so safe right now. Do not be offended if they talk to friends, cousins, and other people besides you about cancer. They may be afraid to really let you know their feelings; it is hard enough to pull things out of teenagers on a regular basis. Continue to be there for them and let them know you are as angry over this as they may be. It might be a good starting point of communication.

People may offer their help in the form of preparing meals, shopping for you, or taking care of things around your house. Some of us find it hard to accept help, but if you need it, accept it. Having a meal made for you on your treatment day may really give you peace of mind because you don't have to worry about cooking.

Some of your close friends may stop talking to you. It's not because they don't care or don't want to know what is going on—it's because they don't know what to say and don't want to make things worse for you. Let friends and family know it is okay to call and talk to you. Sometimes, however, you may have to tell them you don't want to talk about cancer or your treatment at this time, that you just want to hear everyday, normal things.

If you are finding yourself telling your story over and over, it may be time to explain to friends and family that you have been telling this story so many times that you just can't do it right now. You may have to guide some of the conversations. Some people find it helpful to have one other person become the provider of information; other people create a Web site and update it frequently so people can look at this site and write their own notes back to you. Simple email may work, because you can do this in your own time and at your own pace. This is the time to be selfish for you and for your family and to do what works best for *you*.

Some people decide to tell their boss and coworkers about their cancer, whereas some choose to not tell them. This is your decision, but if you need time away from work, you will have to offer some reason. The Americans with Disabilities Act provides you with some job protection, so you should be able to work out a schedule with your boss that will meet your medical needs and at the same time ensure that the work that needs to be done at your job gets completed. You can either explain that you have cancer or simply tell your boss that you are under a doctor's care and that you will need to miss time from work occasionally.

Regardless of how you tell those you love and care about, or what you tell them, follow your heart—it won't lead you wrong. Be patient with yourself and those you are telling; everyone will need time to adjust and settle into the routine of life with cancer and its treatment.

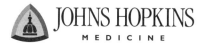

CHAPTER 6

MAINTAINING BALANCE— WORK AND LIFE DURING TREATMENT

H aving cancer is a life-changing event. The moment you are told you have cancer is always a time of deep emotional crisis and distress. This may be the biggest and most frightening challenge. A cancer diagnosis does not mean that your life should come to a halt, but there will be a need for adjustments. You may continue with your daily life and do as much as you can if there is no medical reason to do less than you did before. You and your family should try to maintain as normal a life as possible while you are having treatment.

Recovery from surgery for pancreatic cancer takes time. Adjustments to your diet may occur. Handling a new diagnosis of diabetes along with surgery may need to be addressed. Often a number of therapies for the treatment of pancreatic cancer are given, along with much information about managing side effects. All of these treatments and the sequence in which they may be given may cause concern as to how you will manage your life, including a work schedule. Treatment for pancreatic cancer, however, will be paramount, and your healthcare team is there to help you make adjustments.

ADJUSTING TO YOUR NEW SITUATION

Many patients and their family members have trouble getting used to the role changes that may be required when a loved one has cancer.

MONEY

Cancer treatments and medications can be expensive and can reduce the amount of money your family has to spend or save. If you are not able to work, someone else in your family may need to find a job to help with expenses. You and your family will need to learn more about your health insurance and find out what tests and medications are covered.

LIVING ARRANGEMENTS

When dealing with the treatment for your cancer, you may need to move in with someone else to help with your needed care. This may be difficult because you may feel that you are losing your independence, at least for a little while. If you have to be away from home for treatment, take a few personal effects with you to have something familiar even in a strange place.

DAILY ACTIVITIES

Many patients are used to being independent and accustomed to juggling many activities and duties in their personal lives. You may need help with routine activities, transportation, shopping, cooking, and so on. Asking for and accepting help from others are things you may not feel comfortable doing. Generally, family and friends want to help, and these small tasks are types of things that they can do and that are beneficial to you. Asking others to do things for you may be hard, but it is not a sign of weakness.

If you require chemotherapy, organize a calendar for when your treatments will take place. See if you can arrange your chemotherapy for the end of the week so you can have the weekend to rest and regain your strength. For radiation therapy, consider scheduling the treatments at the very beginning or end of the day. Radiation therapy may be done every day for a number of weeks, so you will want to minimize disruption to your daily routine as much as possible.

You may need someone to accompany you to your treatments, as the day needs to be a relaxed one for you. Consider hiring someone or finding a volunteer through local support groups in your community or church. Try to continue to carry out regular household chores, grocery shopping, or hobbies that you enjoy. It is critical to develop a plan and a schedule that works for both you and those helping you.

MANAGING THE SIDE EFFECTS OF TREATMENT

Make sure you eat something before your treatment, because you need to maintain body weight to fuel your recovery. Prepare or bring a light meal or snack in an insulated bag or small cooler during treatment sessions. If your treatment causes GI (gastrointestinal) side effects, they will usually happen 16 to 48 hours after the infusion of chemotherapy. How you tolerate the first chemotherapy cycle sets the stage for how you will tolerate other cycles using the same medicines. Requesting antinausea medications in advance can prevent GI symptoms.

If you receive radiation therapy, you can anticipate feeling fine until about the last 2 weeks of treatment. At this time you may notice increased fatigue because the doses are cumulative. Give yourself extra time to rest at night and even allow yourself naps in the middle of the day. Try to eat a balanced diet that includes protein (meat, milk, eggs, beans, lentils, and legumes) to boost your energy. Prioritize your activities to conserve energy, doing the most important ones first.

Do not be too hard on yourself if side effects make it hard to eat. Try eating small, frequent meals. Go easy on fried or greasy foods because they can be hard to digest. Be sure to drink plenty of water or liquids each day.

Be sure your doctor or nurse knows about any GI side effects you may be experiencing so they can prescribe effective medicines to control nausea and vomiting or treat diarrhea. Appetite loss is often the first side effect, characterized by a general sensation of not being hungry, feeling full faster than normal, or feeling overwhelmed by a normal portion of food. Although a reduced appetite may seem harmless, it can lead to severe weight loss, dehydration, fatigue, poor immune function, and malnutrition. Make every effort to eat as much as possible, because your nutritional needs are higher than ever when undergoing cancer treatment. Cancer and the treatment for your cancer greatly increases the number of calories required daily. The body needs 1000 or more extra calories every day to build new healthy cells. Therefore, the amount you ate before your diagnosis of cancer has no bearing on what you need during treatment. The value of maintaining an adequate intake of food cannot be overemphasized.

Here are some tips to assist in maintaining adequate food intake when you may be overwhelmed by the thought of food:

- Trick yourself into thinking you are eating small portions. Use a large plate to eat a very small amount of food. This tactic convinces your body and mind that you really are not eating much food. Do not fill a whole plate with food.

- Nibble and graze all day. Do not worry about eating regular meals; just try to eat small bites of food throughout the day.

- Set a timer to remind yourself to eat. When you are not hungry, it is easy to allow 6 or 8 hours to pass without eating or drinking anything. Set a kitchen timer for 60 minutes and eat a few bites when it goes off. Reset the timer and repeat this pattern during the hours that you're awake.

- Keep food out where you can see it. Place bowls of snacks such as peanuts, candies, or dried fruit around the house; eat one or two pieces every time you walk by.

- Sip on a beverage with calories. Hot chocolate, sport drinks, and fruit juices are ways to consume calories throughout the day. Keep juice boxes and drink mixes handy, and be sure to drink them.

- Add nutritional supplements such as Ensure, Boost, or Carnation Instant Breakfast, which are good sources of calories, protein, and carbohydrates. You can also make super shakes with ice cream and these nutritional supplements to increase your caloric intake.

- Use plastic silverware. Some medications may cause a metallic taste in your mouth or alter your taste buds.

Using plastic silverware may help to decrease this taste.

- Avoid nutritional supplements such as guarana, ma huang, or ginseng. These are known stimulants, but the stimulation provided by these supplements has not been proven safe or effective for cancer-treatment fatigue, and the supplements may interact with medications recommended during your treatment.

- Eat your favorite foods. This is not the time to worry about fat or cholesterol. If it sounds good to you, eat it.

MALABSORPTION OF FOOD

The ability of the pancreas to make an adequate amount of enzymes to aid with digestion, particularly of fatty foods, may be compromised by having a pancreatic resection or because of the pancreatic cancer itself. Not having an adequate amount of enzymes can lead to malabsorption (difficulty digesting or absorbing nutrients from food into the bloodstream). Signs and symptoms of malabsorption include the following:

- Vague abdominal discomfort or pain
- Abdominal bloating or distention
- Excessive gas
- Belching
- Diarrhea
- Steatorrhea (fatty or floating stools)
- Weight loss

Replacement pancreatic enzymes may be prescribed to assist in your digestion of food. These enzymes are available in different formulations and dosages. The enzyme preparations are dosed by lipase (an enzyme, or chemical, released by the pancreas for digestion) content but also contain amylase and protease (other enzymes released by the pancreas). Enzymes are started at a low dose and increased if your symptoms do not resolve. The amount of pancreatic enzymes required will vary with the amount of food eaten and may need to be increased with larger meals (for example, two pills with a meal and one with a snack).

The following is useful information for patients on pancreatic enzyme supplements:

- Take enzymes at all meals and snacks.

- Enzymes should be taken whole with liquids.

- Antacids that contain calcium or magnesium can interfere with the effectiveness of the enzymes.

- Taking half of your enzyme dose at the beginning of a meal and the other half toward the end of the meal may improve symptoms.

- Taking certain acid-reducing medications (Pepcid [famotidine], Zantac [ranitidine]) along with the pancreatic enzyme supplement may increase the activity of the enzyme.

- If bloating continues while on the pancreatic enzyme supplement, changing to a different formulation may help.

DELAYED GASTRIC EMPTYING

Delayed gastric emptying (DGE) is also called gastroparesis (*gastro* = stomach, and *paresis* = paralysis). This is a condition that affects the ability of the stomach to empty its contents, but there is no blockage (physical obstruction). Symptoms of DGE are:

- Abdominal distention

- Nausea

- Abdominal fullness very soon after meals

- Unintentional weight loss

- Vomiting

Patients may have DGE after a pancreas resection for cancer such as the Whipple procedure. Supportive measures that your healthcare providers may take include ensuring you take in enough liquids and supplementing your diet with nutrition other than that taken by mouth. You may be given nutrition by an IV or by a feeding tube placed into your stomach or small bowel. People with diabetes are also at risk of experiencing DGE, especially new-onset diabetic patients after pancreas surgery. Good control of your blood sugar is essential.

Medications may be given to help your stomach empty its contents. Your doctor or nurse may order different medications or combinations to find the most effective treatment. If you are able to eat, modification of your diet may be needed. Fatty foods and nondigestible fiber (fresh fruits and vegetables) may be poorly emptied from the GI tract. You may need to eat a low-fat diet and frequent, small meals. Meeting with a dietician for assistance and education may be helpful. An excellent resource is the booklet *Diet and Nutrition: Nutritional Concerns with Pancreatic Cancer* from the Pancreatic Cancer Action Network (PanCAN) (see Chapter 11 for more information about pancreatic cancer resources).

APPETITE STIMULANT

Your doctor or nurse may prescribe an appetite enhancer to promote your hunger. Appetite stimulants are usually reserved for people who have lost more than 10% of their usual body weight or are at risk for malnutrition. These medications may take a few weeks to assist in increasing your appetite, and they may not work for every patient. You will need to work with your doctor or nurse to find the medication that is right for you.

OVERCOMING FATIGUE

Cancer-treatment fatigue is more than just being tired. It is an overpowering sense of exhaustion that is not always relieved by rest. It can be mild, causing you to have less energy to do the things you want to do, or it can be severe, affecting many areas of your life and not allowing you to do basic activities.

Fatigue can even significantly decrease your desire to eat or to prepare basic meals and snacks. Suddenly, walking to the kitchen for a snack is like running a marathon. Left unchecked, this can cause you to go many hours or even whole days with only a few bites of food. This pattern can lead to further malnutrition and dehydration, both of which create a vicious cycle of more fatigue.

The best advice for patients with cancer-treatment fatigue is to eat a balanced diet that includes protein-rich foods such as meats, eggs, cheese, peas, and beans, and to drink 8 to 10 glasses of fluids a day. Preventing malnutrition and dehydration can help keep your baseline energy levels up and provide the body with fuel it needs to maintain basic activities.

INFECTION PREVENTION

There will be days when you can anticipate your white blood cell count will go down in response to having received chemotherapy. This is a period about 10 to 14 days after chemotherapy when you are more vulnerable to getting a cold, flu, or other form of infection. You may want to avoid being in the presence of young children because they can be sick without appearing so. Wearing a mask may be beneficial if you cannot avoid being around children in a closed environment.

Eating a balanced diet that is rich in fruits and vegetables further improves your immune system. It is necessary to wash your hands frequently. You are advised to get a flu shot or to have any dental work done before you start chemotherapy or radiation therapy. If you need to travel by air while undergoing chemotherapy, wear a mask to reduce risk of exposure. In winter, be sure to bundle up and keep warm when outdoors. Your mission is to be healthy during your chemotherapy or radiation treatments and to reduce the risk of exposure to infection as much as possible. Your blood will be drawn periodically to assess how your body's immune system is responding to treatments and whether you need medicine to boost your white blood cell count.

ACCEPTING A CHANGING BODY IMAGE

Weight loss may be initially experienced by a patient with pancreatic cancer. Weight gain from an increase in body fluid, especially in a patient's abdomen (called ascites), may also occur. These changes in body image may present a whole new set of challenges to patients during and even after treatment.

HELPFUL HINTS

Cancer can drain you physically and mentally, but there are ways to bolster your inner reserves. Specifically tailored foods and fitness can ward off fatigue and infection. There is also your psyche or mental health to consider, which is critical in how you approach and deal with your cancer. Here are some useful things to remember.

- *Exercise.* Aerobic exercise can relieve side effects such as depression, decreased appetite, nausea, and fatigue.

- *Skin care.* Cancer treatments may cause changes in your skin. Skin that is normally oily can become temporarily dry and flaky. Your skin tone can change, making you look more ruddy, sallow, or tanned. To keep your skin as healthy as possible, your primary goal is to restore moisture without causing irritation.

- *Nutrition and proper diet.* A proper diet is your ally while undergoing cancer treatment, even if you do not always feel like eating because of nausea, mouth sores, or jaw pain. Your body needs plenty of calories and protein to heal, and the right foods can go a long way toward alleviating fatigue, poor wound healing, and decreased immunity, helping you to bounce back faster once treatment is completed.

KNOWING WHEN TO ASK FOR HELP

There are certain signs that indicate you may need help from your healthcare team. Talk to your doctor, nurse, or social worker if you have any concerns that seem too big to manage on your own or if any of the following occurs:

- You feel overwhelmed, depressed, sad, hopeless, discouraged, or "empty" almost every day, or you have lost interest or pleasure in activities that were once enjoyable.

- You notice extreme changes in your eating habits (eating too much or too little) or have weight loss or gain.

- You have changes in your sleep pattern (inability to sleep, waking too early, or sleeping too much).

- You have feelings of guilt, worthlessness, or hopelessness.

- You have trouble concentrating, remembering, or making decisions.

- You have thoughts of death (not just fear of dying) or suicide, or make attempts at suicide.

- You notice wide mood swings from depression to periods of agitation and high energy.

Cancer treatments may cause some of these symptoms. If these symptoms last for 2 weeks or longer or are severe enough to interfere with your normal functions, an evaluation by a mental health professional may be needed.

RESUMING WORK WHILE RECEIVING TREATMENT

This is a difficult and personal question. Maintaining employment during cancer treatment can be difficult. However, many psychologists feel that maintaining employment is ideal because it helps people to better cope with their disease. The decision to continue working during treatment, whether part time or full time, should be made between you and your doctor. It may depend on how well you feel during treatment and the type of work you do. If you decide to tell your employer about your health, do your homework first. Talk with your doctor about how your treatments may affect your ability to do your job. Then give your employer as much information as necessary about your diagnosis of cancer.

If you require time off from work for treatment, you should consider talking with your employer, so he or she knows why you will be gone from work. There are federal regulations that protect your rights while undergoing treatment—the Americans with Disabilities Act. Employers cannot make you take a physical examination or ask medically related questions unless they concern job performance. Most employers will try to work with you while you are having treatment. It is a good idea to keep careful records of all talks with your employer or with people in the benefits office. Keep copies of your performance reviews. Legal assistance is available if you feel you have been treated unfairly at work. Many companies have a medical leave of absence program or disability leave. Depending on your employer, you either may or may not receive wages during this period. The best part about these leave plans is that they continue your health insurance while you are absent from your job. Telecommuting may also be an option that allows you to work around your treatment schedule. You may want to suggest doing work from your home office when talking to your employer. If you are considering cutting back your hours to a part-time basis, remember that this may affect your benefits.

COPING WITH PANCREATIC CANCER

How you come to terms with the diagnosis of pancreatic cancer is a personal issue. Coping is making decisions, solving problems, and adapting to life's changes while still feeling good about yourself. Factors that affect how well you are able to cope are your emotions, whether you have a positive outlook, and whether you have physical and emotional support.

Many difficult and mixed emotions may come and go over the course of your cancer diagnosis and treatment, including shock, disbelief, fear, anxiety, guilt, sadness, loneliness, depression, grief, and anger. These are normal reactions. You may need to work through these emotions to successfully cope with your diagnosis. Most patients are not prepared for the stresses caused by pancreatic cancer and need to find different ways of handling emotions, thoughts, and behaviors. You may cope better by talking with other people about your emotions, writing in a journal, or taking personal, quiet time.

Making decisions is a large part of dealing with your cancer. Knowing you have some control over what happens to you may make things easier. Learning as much as possible about pancreatic cancer may help you make informed choices, realize you have choices, and then aid in making the best choice for you. It is important for you to focus on things that you can control or change and not on those you cannot.

Having a positive attitude and hoping for the best possible outcome may help you to follow medical advice and take care of yourself physically, mentally, and emotionally. It is advantageous for you to live in the present and focus on what is most important, meaningful, and enjoyable right now, rather than on what you do not have or may lose.

Depression is common in patients with pancreatic cancer. You may have signs and symptoms of depression or anxiety that take over your whole life and cause emotional paralysis. Being depressed is different from being sad. Signs and symptoms to assess include feeling powerless, hopeless, or that you have nothing to live for. These negative feelings may not go away no matter what you do. Family members and friends may notice these emotional changes in you. You or your family members or friends should notify your healthcare team in this case because there are effective medications and other methods available to treat depression.

Some signs and symptoms of depression include the following:

Emotional
- Sadness or a feeling of emptiness
- Loss of interest or pleasure in usual activities
- Feeling guilty, hopeless, or worthless
- Feeling overwhelmed
- Feeling angry or irritable
- Crying often
- Focus on worries and problems
- Inability to concentrate or to make decisions
- Thoughts of death or suicide

Physical
- Difficulty sleeping or sleeping too much
- Feeling tired all the time
- Headaches
- Upset stomach
- Diarrhea
- Dry mouth

RESPECTING THE NEEDS OF YOUR LOVED ONES

Pancreatic cancer treatment creates additional stress for you, your family members, and your friends. Just as you need time for yourself, so too your loved ones need time to rest and to take care of their own responsibilities. It is important for you and your family to design a schedule to best meet your needs—with as little change as possible in your daily routine.

As much as you would like, it is probably not realistic to expect life to be the same as it was before cancer arrived. No matter how you may feel about the treatment, having cancer is still a major crisis. You may have a lot of anxiety about what the future holds. Be aware that life probably will not feel "normal" again for some time. This does not mean that life will be changed forever in a bad way or that your spouse or children's lives will be ruined. Many people say that having cancer resulted in a positive change for their family. People do learn to live, even thrive, with cancer. The challenge is to discover what works best for your own family.

Try to anticipate any changes to your family routines that are needed to deal with unexpected events. Making lists of tasks to be done and assigning each of them to a family member helps life run more smoothly. Regular family meetings can help solve problems before they become huge and relieve tension by airing small concerns. Empower your children to set up meetings whenever they have questions or anxieties of their own.

You can reach out to family and friends for emotional support to help cope with your cancer. Remember, however, that family members may not want to talk because they may be too emotionally involved and do not want to hear what you say. It may be difficult for a loved one to deal with your diagnosis of cancer.

You may be able to express feelings to other patients with cancer that you can't express to your family. Validation of your feelings can come from other patients. Sharing experiences, trading experiences, and giving advice to other people with pancreatic cancer may be beneficial both for you and the other patients. Support groups, individual counseling, and group counseling are ways of communicating to help you cope. Support groups meet in person, by phone, or through reputable Internet sites. Members of your healthcare team should be contacted to discuss anything related to your cancer, your feelings, and how you are coping with it because they are also part of your support system. They can also help find you needed support services.

FINDING MORE TIME AND MODIFYING YOUR PRIORITIES

Most people find it hard to fit everything into their family's schedule even without the demands of cancer and cancer treatment. Cancer and cancer treatment are tough on a physical, emotional, and practical level.

Given all the demands on your time, it can be easy to forget to make time for yourself. *Concentrate on what matters most to you.* Decide which tasks are priorities for you and which tasks you can ask someone else to do or just leave undone. Setting aside time instead to do something you enjoy or just to relax and rest is an important part of the healing and recovery process.

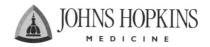

CHAPTER 7

JOHNS HOPKINS
M E D I C I N E

SURVIVING PANCREATIC CANCER— RE-ENGAGING IN MIND AND BODY HEALTH AFTER TREATMENT

Some patients with pancreatic cancer may undergo a course of treatment that eventually ends, whereas other patients may have ongoing cancer treatment. If you are completing a course of treatment, you may find yourself entering a whole new world—one filled with new questions. You are probably relieved and ready to put the experience behind you; yet at the same time, you may feel sad and worried. It is common to be concerned about whether the cancer will come back and what you should do after treatment.

When treatment ends, you may expect life to return to the way it was before you were diagnosed with cancer, but it can take time to recover, and you may never return to your previous life. You may have permanent scars on your body, or you may not be able to do some things you once did easily. You may think that others view you in a different way. One of the hardest things to realize after treatment is that you can't know for sure what will happen next. Those who have gone through cancer treatment describe the first few months as a time of change. It is not so much "getting back to normal" as a time of finding out what is normal for you now. People often say that life has new meaning or that they look at things differently after treatment. Your new "normal" may include making changes in the way you eat, the things you do, and your sources of support. You can also expect things to keep changing as you continue on with your life.

Treatment for pancreatic cancer may be a continuous process for you if you could not have surgery, and you may experience the same issues as just described. In both cases a person may have to deal with the same emotional and physical problems.

EMOTIONAL HEALING

Depending on your stage of pancreatic cancer and the treatment course you take, your emotional state must be considered. Some patients may have continuous treatment with more frequent follow-up visits, whereas others may complete a course of treatment with less frequent follow-up. However, going for checkups often gives patients a sense of security. Some people describe feeling abandoned and a little frightened when they need less frequent follow-up. You may experience worry that the cancer will come back, anger that you are not able to just get on with your life as before, or irritation that the people around you do not understand how you feel.

Your relatives and friends may find your behavior unpredictable or confusing. They may not identify with why you do not feel enthusiastic about getting on with your life. They may be unsure how to respond to you, and you may not know what to say to them. You should develop a wellness plan that includes ways you can address your physical, social, and spiritual needs. If your doctor or nurse, a family member, or a friend recommends that you consider seeing a counselor, do not think you have failed at getting yourself back on track. All of this is hard. Many patients benefit from seeing a counselor to assist them in regaining control or in reengaging in their lives both physically and emotionally. Sometimes, just having a professional sounding board gives perspective to your thoughts and fears. Remember, you are not alone, and what you are experiencing is the norm, not the exception.

MANAGING LONG-TERM SIDE EFFECTS

Side effects from treatment may continue or remain for an extended period of time even after treatment has ended. You may be dealing with changes in bowel function, managing diabetes, alterations in digestion, fatigue, difficulty concentrating, pain, peripheral neuropathy, or any combination of these. It is important to keep in mind that no two people are alike, and your response to therapy and its side effects is unique to you.

CHANGES IN BOWEL FUNCTION

Diarrhea may result from pancreatic cancer or its treatment. This occurs because there is a decrease in the amount of enzymes being produced by the pancreas to assist with digestion. The diarrhea is generally described as frequent soft or more fluid bowel movements. Each person's description of diarrhea is unique based on his or her previous bowel experience.

Pancreatic enzymes may need to be taken with your meals to help digest carbohydrates, protein, and, especially, fats from foods. A discussion with your doctor, nurse, or an oncology dietician can help to evaluate your need for this type of medication.

MANAGING DIABETES

Patients with pancreatic cancer may develop diabetes from the disease or its treatment, particularly as a result of extensive surgery. If you develop diabetes, you will benefit from being evaluated and followed by those healthcare providers who specialize in diabetes management, such as an endocrinologist or a nurse who specializes in diabetes management and education. Patients with diabetes and cancer have special nutritional needs and need to see a dietician for guidance with diabetes medicines, meal schedules, and the added influence of cancer treatment.

ALTERATION IN DIGESTION

Alterations in your digestion of food may result from surgery, chemotherapy, or radiation treatment. Loss of appetite or poor appetite is common in patients with pancreatic cancer. Many patients have problems with weight loss from decreased appetite and feel full after a few bites of food. Abdominal bloating and excess gas are other side effects that may interfere with adequate nutrition and your ability to take in adequate food.

Your nutritional goal should be to eat adequate amounts of fluids, calories, protein, and vitamins to maintain a desirable weight and allow you to continue normal daily activities. Recommendations for dietary intake and avoidance of side effects include the following:

- Eat small, frequent (five to six) meals a day, along with snacks throughout the day.

- At each meal, eat nutritious food and snacks.

- Eat high-calorie foods and whole grains as tolerated.

- Plan to eat your largest meal when most hungry (many patients are most hungry in the morning after a good night's sleep).

- Plan some exercise before eating to help stimulate your appetite.

- Drink liquids about 1 hour before or after eating to avoid a feeling of fullness.

- Drink adequate amounts of fluids to keep yourself hydrated.

- Stay in a sitting position for at least an hour after eating to help avoid heartburn (acid reflux).

- Take antacids (proton pump inhibitors such as Prevacid, Protonix [pantoprazole], etc.) as prescribed to help avoid heartburn.

Meeting with an oncology dietician may be most helpful for dealing with problems with digestion and adequate nutrition intake. An oncology dietician can make recommendations for any dietary changes that may be necessary. The dietician can consult with your doctor or nurse to recommend medications, including pancreatic enzymes, antacids, and medications to help stimulate your appetite.

An excellent source of nutrition information for patients with pancreatic cancer is the booklet *Diet and Nutrition: Nutritional Concerns with Pancreatic Cancer*, available from the Pancreatic Cancer Action Network (http://www.pancan.org).

FATIGUE

Some cancer patients report that they feel tired or worn out. In fact, fatigue is one of the most common complaints for patients with pancreatic cancer. Rest or sleep does not always cure this type of fatigue, and healthcare professionals do not know its exact causes. Fatigue during treatment can be caused by surgery, chemotherapy, radiation, anemia, or a susceptible immune system. Poor nutrition, not drinking enough fluids, and depression all contribute and are further exacerbated by postoperative pain. There is no common pattern as to when fatigue will resolve. For most patients, it simply improves over time.

Potential solutions to help with fatigue include the following:

- Avoid medications that affect your energy level

- Keep pain under good control

- Take part in exercise and relaxation programs

- Change your diet or drink more fluids

- Work with physical and occupational therapists as well as dieticians and mental health counselors

- Plan most of your activities for when you feel most alert

- Take short naps or sleep and wake up at the same time every day

MEMORY AND CONCENTRATION CHANGES

Research shows that one in four people with cancer reports memory and attention problems after chemotherapy, often called "chemo brain." This resembles a brain fog that can lead to difficulties in paying attention, finding the right words, or remembering new concepts. These effects can begin during or after treatment, or they may not appear until much later. They do not always go away. Some patients just cannot focus as they once did.

The following techniques can help heighten memory and concentration:

- *Jot down lists and tasks.* You can write down in a notebook or pocket calendar each task, how long it will take, and where you need to go. Plan your whole day. Keep it simple, and be realistic about how much you can do in a day.

- *Set up reminders.* Put small notes around the house to remind you of things to do, such as taking out the trash or locking the door.

- *Group long numbers.* For example, the phone number 912-5546 can be repeated as "nine-twelve, fifty-five, forty-six."

- *Manage stress.* Managing stress better may improve your memory and attention.

- *Review what you plan to say.* Before you go to family events or work functions, go over names, dates, and key points you want to make.

- *Repeat what you want to remember.* Saying it a couple of times can help your mind hold on to the information.

PAIN

Some people have significant pain from pancreatic cancer even after treatment, whereas others have less. Everyone is different. With your help, your doctor or nurse can assess how severe your pain is and may recommend one or more of the following approaches:

- *Anti-inflammatory medications and narcotics.* In most cases, doctors will try the mildest medicines first. Then you may be given stronger pain medicines if you need them. To keep pain under control, do not skip doses or wait until you have pain to take these medicines.

- *Physical therapy.* The therapist may use heat, cold, massage, pressure, and exercise to make you feel better.

- *Acupuncture.* This is a proven method using needles at specific pressure points to reduce pain.

- *Hypnosis, meditation, or yoga.* Many people have found that practicing deep relaxation relieves or reduces stress.

- *Nerve blocks or surgery.* Nerve blocks or surgery often help if you have persistent or limiting pain.

- *Pain diary.* Use a diary to record and rate your pain to determine whether there are patterns or predisposing factors.

NERVOUS SYSTEM CHANGES (NEUROPATHY)

Occasionally, cancer treatment can cause damage to your nervous system, often referred to as neuropathy. These symptoms can be made worse by other conditions, including diabetes, kidney failure, alcoholism, and malnutrition.

Most people first notice symptoms in their hands and feet, usually starting with their fingertips and toes. Commonly, patients report tingling, burning, weakness, or numbness in hands and feet; sudden, sharp, stabbing, or electric-shock sensations; loss of balance or difficulty walking; clumsiness; trouble picking up objects or buttoning clothes; hearing loss; jaw pain; constipation; and being more or less sensitive to heat and cold. A number of therapies may be tried, including medications, topical creams, pain patches, acupuncture, physical therapy, and exercise.

EVOLVING SEX LIFE

Even if your treatment does not leave significant visible scars, the changes in your body (whether from surgery, chemotherapy, radiation, or the effects of certain medicines) may trouble you. Feeling bad about your body can also lower your sex drive. This loss of reduction in your sex life may add to your grief or depression. Many cancer patients are not prepared for these changes. You may worry about intimacy after treatment. Patients may worry that having sex will hurt or that they will not be able to perform. Discussing your sexual concerns with your doctors and nurses may be beneficial because they can usually answer many of the questions, help correct any underlying medical issues, or assist you in seeing a professional counselor. You may feel that some of your sexual problems are due to your emotions, such as stress, and talking to a sex therapist or psychologist may help.

OPENING UP TO YOUR PARTNER

Even for a couple who has been together for a long time, staying connected can be a major challenge. It may be comforting to learn that very few committed relationships end because of scars or other body changes. Tell your partner how you feel about your sex life and what you would like to change. You may want to talk about your concerns, your beliefs about why your sex life is the way it is, your feelings, and what would make you feel better.

Approaching your sexual concerns honestly avoids blame, keeps things positive, and gives your partner a better sense of how you are feeling. Try to be open-minded as you listen to your partner's point of view:

- Focus on your partner's comments, not on what you plan to say in response.
- Repeat what your partner says in your own words.
- Ask questions to better understand your partner's concerns.
- Acknowledge that your partner's views matter to you.

To increase feelings of intimacy:

- Think of things that help you feel more confident.
- Focus on the positive.

FAITH, RELIGION, OR SPIRITUALITY

Having a serious illness can likewise affect your spiritual outlook. After treatment, you and your loved ones may struggle to understand why you have to endure such a trial in your life. For some, spirituality may get stronger or seem more vital. Others may question their faith and wonder about the meaning of life or their purpose in it. Many say they develop a new focus and try to live each day to the fullest.

Through faith, many cancer patients have been able to find meaning in their lives and make sense of their cancer experience. Religion can be a way for you to connect with others in your community who may share similar experiences. It can also provide an outlet for coping and recovering from cancer. Seeking answers and searching for personal meaning in spirituality can offer hope, perspective, and comfort.

JOINING A SUPPORT GROUP

Support groups can have many benefits. Even though many patients receive support from friends and family, support groups offer opportunities to connect with others who have had similar cancer experiences. Some benefits of a support group are as follows:

- *Sharing of personal stories.* Telling and hearing stories about living with cancer can help people air their concerns, solve problems, or find meaning in what they have been through.

- *Discovery of humor and laughter.* When you laugh, your brain releases chemicals that produce pleasure and relax your muscles. Even a smile can fight off stressful thoughts.

- *Dealing with practical issues.* You can learn how others handle issues at work and how to troubleshoot enduring side effects from treatment.

TYPES OF SUPPORT GROUPS AND WHERE TO FIND THEM

There are many different types of support groups. They may be led by health professionals or fellow cancer survivors, and they are not just for people who have cancer but also for children or other family members. Support groups can meet in person or online. Internet resources can be a big help to people with computers who live in rural areas or who have trouble getting to meetings. With informal chat or discussion groups, you can seek support at any time of the

99

day or night. However, although these online groups can provide valuable emotional support, they may not always provide correct medical information, and you need to be careful about making any changes based on what you read.

IS A SUPPORT GROUP RIGHT FOR ME?

A support group may not be right for everyone. If you are thinking about joining a group, here are some questions you may want to ask the contact person:

- How large is the group?
- Who attends (survivors, family members, types of cancer, age range)?
- How long are the meetings?
- How often does the group meet?
- How long has the group been together?
- Who leads the meetings—a professional or a survivor?
- What is the format of the meetings?
- Is the main purpose to share feelings or offer problem-solving tips?
- If I go, can I just sit and listen?

Before joining a group, here are questions you may want to ask yourself:

- Am I comfortable talking about personal issues?
- Do I have something to offer the group?
- What do I hope to gain by joining a group?

Support groups vary greatly, and if you have one bad experience, it does not mean they are not a good option for you.

Instead, you may want to find another cancer survivor with whom you can discuss your cancer experience. Many organizations can pair you with someone who had your type of cancer and who is close in age or background.

TAKING CHARGE OF YOUR HEALTH

Unfortunately, many patients with pancreatic cancer are never cured of the disease. Patients who have surgery in which all the cancer appears to be removed often have recurrence of their cancer. Newer treatments and combinations of treatments are allowing patients to live longer, however, and even making pancreatic cancer a chronic disease with ongoing treatment.

Keeping up with the latest research published about pancreatic cancer is helpful and empowering. Take measures to regain a personal balance. Eating healthy, exercising, reducing stress, and living as healthy a life as possible enable you to take care of yourself. Taking charge of your health and psychological well-being should be your priority. Some suggestions follow:

- *Be informed.* Learning about your cancer, understanding what you can do for your health now, and finding out about the services available can give you a greater sense of control. Several studies suggest that people who are well informed about their illness and treatment are more likely to follow their treatment plans and to handle their cancer diagnosis and treatment better than those who are uninformed.

- *Express your feelings of fear, anger, or sadness.* People have found that when they express strong feelings such as anger or sadness, they are more able to let go of them. Some sort out their feelings by writing then down or talking to friends, family, or other cancer survivors.

- *Concentrate on staying healthy.* Occasionally, this means looking for the good even in a bad time or trying to be hopeful instead of thinking the worst. Direct your energy to staying as healthy as possible.

- *Don't blame yourself for your cancer.* Some people believe that they got cancer because of something they did or did not do. Remember, cancer can happen to anyone.

- *Find ways to help yourself relax.* Spend quiet time at home or at a café, or simply get out of the house; this can help you focus on other things besides cancer and the worries it brings.

- *Look at what you can control.* Being involved in your health care, keeping your appointments, and making active lifestyle changes gives you a sense of control.

SEEING THE WORLD THROUGH DIFFERENT EYES

Take time to step back and reassess your life. What you thought was important before may have little meaning now. Consider setting short-term and long-term goals. These goals may be directed at living your life to the fullest each day, or you may be focused on how you want to make a difference for others who are diagnosed with this disease. You are truly connected to an extraordinary group of people—patients who share common thoughts, dreams, and fears.

Whether willingly or not, your cancer has changed you, and you should value every day and every encounter as a new opportunity to grow and achieve personal happiness.

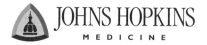

CHAPTER 8

MANAGING RISK—WHAT IF MY CANCER COMES BACK?

The risk of recurrence remains the most feared issue that patients may deal with when they have finished their treatment for pancreatic cancer. Learning what to look for, when and how to look for it, and for how long is helpful. Putting the risk of recurrence in perspective is extremely important to your psychological well-being.

PREVENTION AND MONITORING FOR RECURRENCE

Despite the development of more sophisticated diagnostic techniques, pancreatic cancer is not detected in its early stages. Surgery for pancreatic cancer offers the only likelihood of cure. Long-term survival is observed in only a small group of patients. The 5-year survival rate for a patient who has had a Whipple procedure for pancreatic cancer is 10% to 20%, although in highly selected patients with localized cancer that has not spread to the lymph nodes, median survival can approach 50% at 5 years. Most patients, however, will develop recurrent disease within 2 years after curative treatment. This usually occurs either at the site of resection, in the liver, or on the surface of the organs in the abdomen. Chemotherapy, with or without radiation therapy, after surgery has shown early encouraging results in prolonging survival in patients with metastatic pancreatic cancer, and radiation therapy may also be used occasionally for symptom relief in recurrent disease. Surgery has a limited role in the treatment of recurrence except in highly selected circumstances for management of symptoms such as bowel obstruction.

It is now known that micro-metastases, or microscopic cancer cells, stay in the body even after all visible cancer has been removed in surgery. Even the most advanced CT scans or MRIs may not detect early recurrence of pancreatic cancer. Recurrence may be suspected when the level of the cancer marker CA 19-9 starts to rise. Other symptoms that may occur include pain, weight loss, lack of appetite, and an increase in abdominal girth known as ascites.

Although data on the role of surveillance in patients with resected pancreatic cancer are limited, the earlier the recurrent disease is identified, the sooner you may be eligible for treatment with standard chemotherapy or to qualify for a clinical trial. The National Comprehensive Cancer Network (NCCN) guidelines suggest the following schedule for follow-up visits:

- History and physical examination for symptom assessment every 3 to 6 months for 2 years

- CA 19-9 level assessment and CT scans every 3 to 6 months for 2 years

A medical oncologist or surgical oncologist usually provides this follow-up care. If there is no evidence of recurrence after 5 years of follow-up, you may be followed then by your primary care provider.

Although the opportunity to extend survival is greatest before the cancer has spread, treatment also can help to control symptoms and complications in the later stages of the disease.

WHAT HAPPENS WHEN THE CANCER COMES BACK?

A variety of factors ultimately influence a patient's decision about whether to receive treatment for recurrent pancreatic cancer. The purpose of receiving cancer treatment may be to improve symptoms through local control of the cancer or to prolong survival. The potential benefits of receiving cancer treatment must be carefully balanced with the potential risks of treatment. The following is a general overview of the treatment of recurrent pancreatic cancer. Circumstances unique to your situation and the prognostic factors of your cancer may ultimately influence how these general treatment principles are applied.

For most patients, recurrent pancreatic cancer is incurable with the currently available standard therapies. Pancreatic cancer may recur locally or spread to other organs such as the liver or lungs, or to the abdomen.

LOCAL RECURRENCE

If the recurrence of the pancreatic cancer is located only in the area of the surgery (where the pancreas was cut), without evidence of cancer anywhere else in the body, enrollment in a clinical trial is preferred. Chemotherapy along with radiation therapy may be considered. The total dose of radiation therapy given before surgery will need to be considered to see if any further radiation can be given safely. Supportive care is always an option to be considered.

METASTATIC DISEASE

When the cancer recurs outside of the pancreas, several treatment options could be considered. The treatment options depend on your health status and the treatment received at the time of the initial diagnosis.

Radiation therapy along with chemotherapy may be considered in the setting of uncontrolled pain due to local recurrence as well as for metastatic disease if these therapies had not been given previously. If your pain is under control, then systemic chemotherapy would be given. If the pancreatic cancer has metastasized in less than 6 months following completion of primary therapy, you may want to consider a clinical trial or you could switch to another line of systemic chemotherapy. If the pancreatic cancer has spread more than 6 months after completion of primary therapy, a clinical trial may also be appropriate. Sometimes, in this setting, it may be reasonable to get retreated with the systemic therapy that was previously given. In either time frame, supportive therapy may be recommended depending on your particular situation.

CLINICAL TRIALS

Before starting treatment, you may want to think about taking part in a clinical trial. Information about clinical trials can be found in Chapter 3.

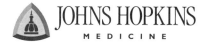

CHAPTER 9

MY CANCER ISN'T
CURABLE—WHAT NOW?

BY MARIAN GRANT, DNP, CRNP, ACHPN

ADDITIONAL SERVICES AND TREATMENT OPTIONS

From the beginning of your illness, you may have had a number of physical and emotional issues. Perhaps it was physical symptoms that led to your diagnosis. Or perhaps you were feeling fine before but now that you've received the diagnosis, you're having a hard time dealing with it. Sometimes there can be discomfort from the treatments for cancer, such as chemotherapy or radiation. If you had surgery, you may have some trouble recovering from that. You need relief and you want to feel better.

You also may want to better understand your situation and choices regarding treatment, and you need to be able to carry on with everyday life. Your healthcare team will probably be the first stop for dealing with any problems with your illness. But, if you need more than your healthcare team can provide, there are other experts who can help. This chapter reviews the possible needs that people with pancreatic cancer have and what and who may be able to help with them.

PHYSICAL DISCOMFORT

Pain

Some people with pancreatic cancer have pain. This can be from surgery or from the cancer pressing on nerves or other internal organs. Pain can come and go or be there all the time. Although this can be distressing and uncomfortable, the good news is that most pain can be controlled. You should keep track of when the pain happens and how long it lasts. Your healthcare team will ask you about that and also about how bad it is, probably using a scale from 1 to 10. Don't worry if you can't answer these questions—they're just a starting point.

There are a number of medicines that can be used for pain, depending on where it is and how often it comes. These may be things you can buy in the drugstore or they may be stronger and need a prescription. Your healthcare team will work with you to find medicines that are appropriate for you. Some of them may have side effects, such as constipation, but most of these side effects can be treated. You should take the pain medicine as directed and let your healthcare team know if you're having any problems.

For pain that can't be controlled with medicines that are taken orally (by mouth), there are other options. Sometimes people need to have the nerves that are in pain "blocked" so that the pain stops. Other people may need to have pain medicine pumps placed under the skin to give a little medicine all the time. Anesthesia pain specialists deal with the management of pain, and you may benefit from seeing these doctors. Again, your healthcare team will work with you if those options are necessary.

Nausea and Vomiting

Nausea and vomiting can happen if the cancer is pressing on parts of the stomach or intestines, or can be side effects from chemotherapy or other medicines. Sometimes changing your diet or taking pancreatic enzyme supplements can help. There are also special medicines that can help with nausea from the cancer or chemotherapy. Let your healthcare team know if this is a problem for you.

Loss of Appetite or Weight

Appetite and weight loss can be related to the problems discussed previously and are not unusual in people who have cancer. Sometimes the problem is that you are eating less because of nausea or pain in your abdomen. Chemotherapy and some medicines can change your sense of taste and make food taste less good. Again, there are changes in diet that can sometimes help, including trying high-calorie supplements to regain weight. Your healthcare team may have experience with this or can refer you to a dietician you can talk with to develop the right diet plan for you. There are also medicines that can help with appetite if diet changes don't work.

Constipation

Constipation is common in patients taking pain medications or those who have some kind of cancer in their abdomen. Typically, you should try whatever you have done in the past for constipation that has worked. However, if your usual remedies or over-the-counter medicines don't help, let your healthcare team know. Make sure you get enough to drink, since dehydration can also lead to constipation. Walking and moving around also helps if you have enough energy.

Diarrhea

Diarrhea can result from changes in your digestive enzymes from the pancreatic cancer. It can also be a result of medicines, such as antibiotics. Talk to your healthcare team if you have this problem so that they can either suggest supplemental pancreatic enzymes or something else for the diarrhea.

Jaundice

Jaundice occurs when the bile that normally flows out of your gallbladder gets blocked by the cancer and starts to build up in your body. It can make your skin and the whites of your eyes yellow. It can also make your urine very dark and change the color of your stool. Many blockages can be corrected by putting a stent into the bile duct to prop it open. Sometimes further surgery is necessary to solve the problem. Jaundice usually isn't uncomfortable, but can sometimes cause you to itch.

Blood Clots

Cancer changes the thickness of your blood, and this can sometimes cause blood clots. Usually these start in the legs, where they can cause swelling, pain, or tenderness. If you notice this, let your healthcare team know right away because blood clots can move up from the legs into the lungs and cause breathing problems. If you develop blood clots, you may need to take blood thinner medications, which will also make you more likely to bleed if you bump or cut yourself.

Ascites

Ascites is fluid that builds up and makes your abdomen become bigger and swollen. It's caused by changes in blood circulation from the cancer. This is usually a sign of the last stages of pancreatic cancer. The fluid and swelling are uncomfortable and can make it hard to breathe. Treatment for this can include water pills to try to get the fluid out through your urine. If that doesn't work, your healthcare team can put a thin needle into the fluid and draw some of it out. This isn't uncomfortable, but may need to be done several times, because the fluid tends to come back.

Fatigue

Fatigue is common in people with cancer. You may be able to do less than before the cancer, which can be hard to accept. Try to get as much rest as possible. If you have problems sleeping, let your healthcare team know because they can suggest things that can help. You may also be tired from having fewer red blood cells, which can happen with some cancer treatment. Again, there are medicines to treat this. Finally, there are special medicines for fatigue, so work with your healthcare team if this is an issue.

Hair Loss and Mouth and Skin Sores

Hair loss, mouth sores, and skin sores can be side effects from chemotherapy. Your healthcare team should be able to tell you whether the drugs you are taking may cause these problems as well as how to treat them. These side effects can be distressing physically and emotionally and make you feel self-conscious.

EMOTIONAL ISSUES

Many people with cancer have emotional issues, and treating them is as important as treating any physical discomfort. It can be hard for someone who's never been depressed or afraid or anxious before to deal with these feelings. Getting a diagnosis of pancreatic cancer can be a very frightening thing. Your feelings may shift back and forth and be unpredictable. Fortunately, there are options to help if these feelings are getting in your way. Some common emotional issues are discussed here.

Depression

Depression can be caused by a combination of things. Perhaps you were already having problems with depression before getting cancer, or perhaps it was having this disease that caused you to feel hopeless. You may be having physical discomfort that can make your mood worse. Or it could be a combination of all three.

Signs of depression can go from feeling unmotivated or down to feeling like life isn't worth living. You may find yourself crying more easily or not finding pleasure in things you used to love. You may be irritable and short-tempered with your loved ones. You may lose your appetite and either sleep too much or too little.

Dealing with a diagnosis of pancreatic cancer is hard, and you may need help to do that. Needing help isn't a bad thing or a sign of weakness. There are a range of actions that can help, such as talking to loved ones or a pastor or spiritual advisor, talking to your healthcare team, writing your thoughts down in a journal, talking to other people with cancer or going online to one of the pancreatic cancer Web sites, and getting involved with activities you love. If doing these things doesn't make your mood better, you should talk to your healthcare team about other treatments. They may suggest counselors to talk to or even medicines to take.

Anxiety

Anxiety is a feeling of fear, helplessness, or panic. It can happen along with depression or on its own. Certainly, there are things to be worried about with pancreatic cancer. However, these feelings may become overwhelming to the point where you need help.

Again, some of the things that help with depression can help with anxiety: talking to others, doing things you love, writing your fears down. In addition, there are medications that can help. Let your healthcare team know if this is a problem for you. They will want to help.

OTHER ISSUES

In addition to physical and emotional problems from cancer, there can be other concerns that cause distress. Pancreatic cancer can affect younger people, and so you may have children you are caring for or may have problems working. You may suddenly go from being a healthy person in the prime of your life to being a patient who is sick. You may have financial concerns over medical expenses, insurance, or loss of income. Your cancer or treatment may make you look different and make you feel self-conscious. Finally, you may need your loved ones to care for you in new ways and may be worried about becoming a burden.

For many people, an illness like pancreatic cancer makes him or her wonder about life, death, God, and meaning. Why did this happen? What will come next? You may find yourself being angry at the situation, and this may cause problems with your loved ones. These are all normal reactions, but can be troublesome. Again, your healthcare team should have resources to help you deal with them. You may find that a friend or spiritual counselor can be of great help. Or, if you're not the kind to talk about these things, you may find books or information online that can help.

If your healthcare team doesn't have the resources to help with these things, you might consider asking for referral to a palliative care specialist. The goal of palliative care is to relieve the pain, symptoms, and stress of serious illness, whatever the diagnosis or prognosis. It is appropriate for people of any age and at any point in an illness. It can be delivered along with treatments that are meant to cure you. Palliative care is typically provided by a team that includes palliative care doctors, nurses, and social workers. The team works in partnership with your healthcare team. If you're in the hospital, there may be a palliative care team that can see you there. Or, there may be a palliative care service at your clinic or medical center. Your healthcare team can connect you to these resources if you need them.

WHAT ARE YOUR TREATMENT GOALS?

This may seem an obvious question, but there are several options, so it helps to think about each of them. Your healthcare team needs to know what your treatment goals are so they can choose the best treatments to achieve them. You should not assume that your goals are obvious. Everyone is different, and it is best to make your goals clear from the start.

Although there are many possible variations, most goals fall into three broad areas: cure, prolonging life, and palliation or comfort. Of course, being comfortable is something to aim for in all three areas. People's goals can change throughout an illness. This is normal, and your healthcare team can help. Communication is key, so feel free to ask any questions and bring up any issues that are important to you. It's also important in thinking about your goals to recognize that any treatment has pros and cons. The treatment might cure or slow the cancer, but it may come with side effects. The side effects may be tolerable or not. It is helpful to assess throughout treatment whether the benefits are worth the side effects. This may change over time. Here are more specifics for each area.

> *Cure.* Some people find that their pancreatic cancer is curable. This is likely through a combination of surgery, chemotherapy, and radiation. Others find that although their cancer is not curable, it is treatable. The two things are not the same. Cancer that is curable will go away after treatment and likely not come back. Cancer that is treatable may shrink or slow with treatment, but will not go away and over time will increase. Often it is difficult to know what will happen with your cancer until you try some treatment. After treatment it may be clearer whether the cancer has been cured or just slowed. You should try to clarify with your healthcare team which category they think you and your cancer fall into and make sure that they keep you updated as time goes along.
>
> Even if your healthcare team thinks your cancer is likely not curable, you may still have this as your goal. Most people hope that their cancer can be cured.

Prolonging life. Even if your cancer is not curable, you may still want to get treatment to prolong your life. Depending on the cancer and the treatment, this could mean a matter of days, weeks, months, or even years. Again, the treatment comes with side effects and thus, it's important to talk with your healthcare team about how much time it is possible to gain versus what the side effects are. Some people are willing to get any treatment that will prolong their lives, even if only for a few days. Others decide that the quality of the time they might gain is not worth the side effects. This is an individual decision and should be made by you, your loved ones, and your healthcare team.

Palliation or comfort. If your cancer is not curable or treatment is not possible or desirable, the option exists of just focusing on keeping comfortable. This could include stopping treatment, deciding not to go to the hospital any more, or getting hospice involved. Hospice is discussed in greater length later in this chapter. This is sometimes a hard choice to make. Usually it comes about after several treatments and discussions with your healthcare team. Families may need to give the person with cancer permission to stop treatment that either isn't working or is causing too much discomfort. It is hard to agree to let loved ones go, and people may need help and support to do that. Your healthcare team can help.

HOPE FOR THE BEST, BUT PLAN FOR THE WORST

Whatever your treatment goals or the stage of your cancer, it can help to plan for what your loved ones should do if you were to become too ill to speak for yourself. (Actually, this is something everyone should do, whether they have cancer or not, since anyone can get sick or be in an accident.) These are difficult things to think and talk about, and some people are not comfortable doing it, which is okay. Others find it comforting to plan for the worst, which is okay, too. Hopefully, the worst won't happen, but if it does, here are things to think about.

Power of Attorney for Healthcare Decisions

The most important thing to do is to pick someone who can make your healthcare decisions in case you are too sick to do so. This person can also have the power of attorney for your financial affairs, but that's a separate process. Ideally, you should talk with the person you pick so that he or she knows what you would want in case you become very ill. Things to discuss are what to do if your heart stops (whether to try CPR or not), what to do if you become so ill you need machines to keep you alive, and how aggressive or long you would want treatment to be if it meant you wouldn't be able to recover fully.

Advance Directives

If you have picked someone as your healthcare proxy and made decisions about these things, you can summarize them in paperwork called advance directives, or a living will. These are legal documents, but you don't need a lawyer to do them. An easy way to do this is to fill paperwork out at the clinic or hospital, where it can be witnessed by someone on the staff. Another option is something called "Five Wishes," which you can download for a small fee from the Internet at http://www.agingwithdignity.org/5wishes.html.

Having things in writing is a good idea, but if you don't get around to filling out the paperwork, you should at least try to tell someone what you would want. We know that loved ones find it easier to make difficult decisions when they know the patient's wishes. That's a gift you can give to them. You should also tell your healthcare team what your wishes are, perhaps when you discuss your treatment goals. They can note your thoughts on these things in your medical chart so that there's a record.

WHEN CANCER TREATMENT IS NO LONGER AN OPTION

Unfortunately, some people may come to a point at which there either isn't any more treatment for their cancer or the treatment is too difficult for their bodies to tolerate. Usually, this happens in the last stages of the disease. It's at this point that hospice may be appropriate.

Hospice is a group of services paid for by insurance or Medicare for people who have less than 6 months to live. The services cover all medicines and medical equipment, and the goal is to make you and your loved ones as physically and emotionally comfortable as possible. These services can be provided in your home, in which case a nurse or aide comes out several times a week to check on you and help your loved ones with any care you may need. It also can be provided in a hospital, a long-term care facility, or a nursing home.

Many people are reluctant to sign up for hospice because it feels like they are giving up. However, we now know that some people actually live longer with hospice care because someone is checking on them regularly and making sure that small problems don't become bigger ones. If you live longer than 6 months, you can continue hospice if your doctor feels that's still the right care for you. If you have any questions about hospice, you can ask your healthcare team or even call a local hospice for more information. They are very supportive, and you may find it helpful to get information in advance of when you might need these services. You can also talk to your healthcare team about hospice at any time.

Even if you don't feel hospice is right for you, you might want to think about what you want to do with whatever time you have left. Some people want to visit a special place or people they love. Others want to spend time at home or with friends in their communities. Most of us have business to put in order, and this can be the time to try to do that.

THE LAST DAYS

People who die from pancreatic cancer, or any kind of cancer, can die from a number of different complications. In the case of pancreatic cancer, patients may become unable to tolerate food in their stomachs and so become weak and prone to infections. If the cancer spreads, it can go into the liver and cause it to stop working properly. It can also spread to the intestines and cause blockages.

Your healthcare team will be committed to trying to handle any medical problems and keeping you comfortable. Whether the team caring for you is a medical team in a hospital or hospice at home, they will try to keep you pain-free, clean, dry, and comfortable. They will talk with your loved ones about what to expect and help with any information on things such as funeral arrangements. Again, some people find it too painful to think of these things in advance, whereas others want to participate in any planning. You will know what's right for you and your loved ones.

Additional resources can be found on the following Web sites:

> GetPalliativeCare.org (http://www.getpalliativecare.org): A Web site about palliative care with information about palliative care in general and also information specific to your location.

> Hospice Net (http://www.hospicenet.org): A Web site full of information on hospice and what services are available in your area.

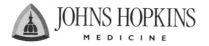

CHAPTER 10

PANCREATIC CANCER IN OLDER ADULTS

By Gary R. Shapiro, MD

Most cases of pancreatic cancer occur in older people, with incidence peaking from age 70 to 80 years. As we live longer, the number of people with cancers of the pancreas will increase. In the next 25 years, the number of people who are 65 years of age and older will double, and the largest increases in cancer incidence will occur in those older than 80 years of age.

Older adults with cancer often have other chronic health problems and may be taking multiple medications that can affect their cancer treatment plan. Prejudice, misunderstanding, and limited access to clinical trials often prevent older patients from getting the timely cancer treatment that they need.

Older men and woman may not have an adequate workup for pancreatic cancer, and when a cancer is found, it is too often ignored or undertreated. Despite the fact that older patients often have early-stage disease, they usually do not undergo pancreatic surgery. As a result, they often have worse outcomes than younger patients. Older people also receive less chemotherapy and less radiation therapy, and their advanced pancreatic cancer is often left untreated.

WHY IS THERE MORE CANCER IN OLDER PEOPLE?

The organs in our body are made up of cells, which divide and multiply as the body needs them. Cancer develops when cells in a part of the body grow out of control. The body has a number of ways of repairing damaged control mechanisms, but as we get older, these do not work as well. Although our healthier lifestyles have allowed us to avoid death from infection, heart attack and stroke, we may now live long enough for a cancer to develop. People who live longer have increased exposure to cancer-causing agents (carcinogens) in the environment, such as tobacco, red meat, and other dietary risks. They are also more likely to be overweight or have diseases like diabetes that increase the risk for developing pancreatic cancer (see Chapter 1). Aging decreases the body's ability to protect us from these carcinogens and to repair cells that are damaged by these and other processes.

PANCREATIC CANCER IS DIFFERENT
IN OLDER PEOPLE

Older people are more likely to present with potentially curable early stage pancreatic cancer than their younger counterparts and, with advancing age, more women are diagnosed. There appear to be no differences in the grade or location (head, body, or tail) of cancers in older versus younger individuals, and no difference in the incidence of local spread. However, some studies have shown that pancreatic cancers cells are less aggressive and less likely to spread through the blood than those of younger patients.

DECISION MAKING: 7 PRACTICAL STEPS

1. GET A DIAGNOSIS

No matter how typical the signs and symptoms, first impressions are sometimes wrong. That suspicious pancreatic mass may not be an adenocarcinoma, but an endocrine tumor that, though malignant, requires relatively simple treatment. It might even be benign. A diagnosis helps you and your family understand what to expect and how to prepare for the future, even if you cannot get curative treatment. Knowing the diagnosis also helps your doctor treat your symptoms better. Many people find not knowing very hard and are relieved when they finally have an explanation for their symptoms. Sometimes a frail patient is obviously dying and diagnostic studies can be an additional burden. In such cases, it may be quite reasonable to focus on symptom relief, or palliation without knowing the details of the diagnosis especially when imaging studies show a "typical" pancreatic mass associated with a high CA 19-9 cancer marker in the blood.

2. KNOW THE CANCER'S STAGE

The cancer's stage defines your prognosis and treatment options. No one can make informed decisions without it. Just as there may be times when the burdens of diagnostic studies may be too great, it may also be appropriate to do without full staging in a very frail, dying patient.

As it is in younger patients, stage is determined by the size of the cancer, the presence or absence of cancer in lymph nodes, or its spread (metastasis) to other organs. When doctors combine this information with information regarding your cancer's site of origin and tissue type (exocrine adenocarcinoma vs. endocrine pancreatic cancers), they can predict what impact, if any, your pancreatic cancer is likely to have on your life expectancy and quality of life.

3. KNOW YOUR LIFE EXPECTANCY

Anticancer treatment should be considered if you are likely to live long enough to experience symptoms or premature death from pancreatic cancer. If your life expectancy is so short that the cancer will not significantly affect it, there may be no reason to treat your cancer. However, chronological age should not be the only thing that decides how your cancer should, or should not, be treated. Despite advanced age, people who are relatively well often have a life expectancy that is longer than their life expectancy with pancreatic cancer. The average 70-year-old woman is likely to live another 16 years, and the average 70-year-old man another 12 years. A similar 85-year-old can expect to live an additional 5 to 6 years, and remain independent for most of that time. Even an unhealthy 75-year-old man or woman probably will live 5 to 6 more years; long enough to suffer symptoms and early death from recurrent pancreatic cancer.

4. UNDERSTAND THE GOALS

The Goals of Treatment

It is important to be clear whether the goal of treatment is cure (surgery with our without adjuvant chemotherapy or radiation therapy) or palliation (radiation or chemotherapy for incurable locally advanced or metastatic pancreatic cancer). If the goal is palliation, you need to understand if the treatment plan will extend your life, control your symptoms, or both. How likely is it to achieve these goals, and how long will you enjoy its benefits?

When the goal of treatment is palliation, chemotherapy should never be administered without defined endpoints and timelines. It should be clear to everyone what counts as success, how it will be determined (for example, a symptom controlled or a smaller mass on CT scan), and when. You and your family should understand what your options are at each step, and how likely each is to meet your goals. If this is not clear, ask your doctor to explain it in words that you understand.

The Goals of the Patient

In addition to the traditional goals of tumor response, increased survival, and symptom control, older cancer patients often have goals related to quality of life. These may include having physical and intellectual independence, spending quality time with your family, taking trips, staying out of the hospital, or even maintaining economic stability. At times, palliative care or hospice may meet these goals better than active anticancer treatment. In addition to the healthcare team, older patients often turn to family, friends, and clergy to help guide them.

5. DETERMINE IF YOU ARE FIT OR FRAIL

Deciding how to treat cancer in someone who is older requires a thorough understanding of his or her general health and social situation. Decisions about cancer treatment should never focus on age alone.

Age Is Not a Number

Your actual age has limited influence on how cancer will respond to therapy or its prognosis. Biological and other changes associated with aging are more reliable in estimating an individual's vigor, life expectancy, or the risk of treatment complications. These changes include malnutrition, depression, dementia, falls, social isolation; and the loss of muscle mass and strength, and the ability to accomplish daily activities such as dressing, bathing, eating, shopping, housekeeping, and managing one's finances or medication.

Chronic Illnesses

Older cancer patients are likely to have chronic illnesses (comorbidity) that affect their life expectancy; the more you have, the greater the effect. This effect has very little impact on the behavior of the cancer itself, but studies do show that comorbidity has a major impact on treatment outcome and its side effects.

6. BALANCE BENEFITS AND HARMS

Fit, older pancreatic cancer patients respond to treatment similarly to their younger counterparts. However, a word of caution is in order. Until recently, few studies included older individuals, and it may not be appropriate to apply these findings to the diverse group of older cancer patients. The side effects of cancer treatment are never less in the elderly. In addition to the standard side effects, there are significant age-related toxicities to consider. Though most of these are more a function of frailty than chronological age, even the fittest senior cannot avoid the physical effects of aging. In addition to the changes in fat and muscle that you see in the mirror, there are age-related changes in your kidney, liver, and digestive (gastrointestinal) function.

These changes affect how your body absorbs and metabolizes anticancer drugs and other medicines. The average senior takes many different medicines (to control, for example, high blood pressure, high cholesterol, osteoporosis, diabetes, arthritis, etc.). This polypharmacy (many drugs) can cause undesirable side effects as the many drugs interact with each other and the anticancer medications.

7. GET INVOLVED

Healthcare providers and family members often underestimate the physical and mental abilities of older people and their willingness to face chronic and life-threatening conditions. Studies clearly show that older patients want detailed and easily understood information about potential treatments and alternatives. Patients and families may consider cancer untreatable in the aged, and, as a result, may not understand the possibilities offered by treatment.

While patients with dementia pose a unique challenge, they are frequently capable of participating in goal setting and simple discussions about treatment side effects and logistics. Caring family members and friends are often able to share the patient's life story so that healthcare workers can work with them to make decisions consistent with the patient's values and desires. This of course is no substitute for a well thought out and properly executed living will or healthcare proxy.

While it is hard to face the possibility of life-threatening events at any age, it is always better to be prepared and to put your affairs in order. In addition to estate planning and wills, it is critical that you outline your wishes regarding medical care at the end of your life and make legal provisions for someone to make those decisions for you if you are unable to make them for yourself.

TREATING PANCREATIC CANCER

YOU NEED A TEAM

Cancer care changes rapidly and it is hard for the generalist to keep up to date, so referral to a specialist is essential. The needs of an older cancer patient often extend beyond the doctor's office and the traditional services provided by visiting nurses. These needs may include transportation or nutrition, and emotional, financial, physical, or spiritual support. When an older woman or man with pancreatic cancer is the primary caregiver for a frail or ill spouse, grandchildren, or other family members, special attention is necessary to provide for their needs as well. Older cancer patients cared for in geriatric oncology programs benefit from multidisciplinary teams of oncologists, geriatricians, psychiatrists, pharmacists, physiatrists, social workers, nurses, clergy, and dieticians, all working together as a team to identify and manage the stressors that can limit effective cancer treatment.

SURGERY

Though pancreatic cancer surgery (see Chapter 3) is complex, it is the standard of care for most early stage cancers of the pancreas, regardless of age. It is the only potentially curative approach for pancreatic cancer. Like other treatment options, surgery in some older individuals may involve risks related to decreases in body organ function (especially heart and lung), and it is essential that the surgeon and anesthetist work closely with your primary care physician (or a consultant) to fully assess and treat these problems before, during, and after the operation. Improvements in surgical techniques now allow Whipple procedures in fit elderly patients without excess mortality, even in those over age 80 years.

As in younger patients, cure rates are low and depend on the stage of the cancer, histology, grade, and the number of lymph nodes affected by the cancer. Surgery is as effective in elderly patients as in younger patients, but it does have a somewhat higher rate of complications in older individuals, especially those over 80, who have other medical problems, or comorbidities. Delayed gastric emptying is a complication of pancreatic cancer surgery, and older patients are at particular risk for resultant malnutrition and dehydration. They also have an increased likelihood of developing diabetes after a distal pancreatectomy or total pancreatectomy, especially if they already have non-insulin diabetes. For patients who have undergone surgical resection, adjuvant radiation and chemotherapy are often given in an attempt to prolong survival (see Chapter 3).

Frail patients or those with inoperable pancreatic cancers or jaundice often benefit from having a stent placed into the obstructed bile duct to help keep it open. As discussed in Chapter 3, this is a nonsurgical palliative treatment that is accomplished by either ERCP or PBD techniques. Surgical bypass procedures (see pages 49–50) are also useful in palliating symptoms due to biliary or gastric outlet obstruction in patients with locally or regionally advanced pancreatic cancer.

RADIATION THERAPY

Radiation therapy may control symptoms and extend life in patients with unresectable pancreatic cancer, but, as discussed in Chapter 3, its use as a single cancer treatment is controversial. It is probably more effective when given with concurrent chemotherapy, but only the fittest people 80 years of age and older are able to tolerate this type of intensive combination therapy.

Older patients are particularly susceptible to nausea, vomiting, diarrhea, loss of appetite, and other side effects from abdominal radiation therapy. Dehydration, weight loss, and electrolyte disturbances can be avoided with careful monitoring and early treatment. Feeding tubes help patients receiving abdominal radiation therapy and chemotherapy get adequate fluid and nutritional support.

The fatigue that usually accompanies radiation therapy can be quite profound in the elderly, even in those who are fit. Often the logistical details, such as daily travel to the hospital for a 6–8 week course of treatment, are the hardest for older people. It is important that you discuss these potential problems with your family and social worker prior to starting radiation therapy.

Bone metastases and spinal cord compression are not as common with pancreatic cancer as with other types of cancer, but if these problems do develop, radiation therapy is usually quite effective palliation for the associated pain and debility. In these situations, a short course of radiation therapy often allows patients with advanced cancer to lower, or even eliminate, their dose of narcotic pain relievers. Although these medicines do an excellent job of controlling pain, they often cause confusion, falls, and constipation in older patients. Thus, even hospice patients suffering from localized metastatic bone pain should consider the option of palliative radiation therapy.

A celiac plexus nerve block is another excellent option for control of the localized abdominal or back pain that is common in patients with pancreatic cancer. It is performed either at the time of surgery or percutaneously, and often relieves one's pain for up to 6 months. Older patients with comorbid diseases may be more susceptible to hypotensive (low blood pressure) side effects, but this type of nerve block is generally quite safe, and, usually allows patients to decrease the amount of narcotics they use; thus, diminishing the side effects (confusion, lethargy, falls, constipation, etc.) of these drugs.

CHEMOTHERAPY

Nonfrail older cancer patients respond to chemotherapy (see Chapter 3) similarly to younger patients. Reducing the dose of chemotherapy or radiation therapy based purely on chronological age may seriously affect the effectiveness of treatment. Managing chemotherapy-associated toxicity with appropriate supportive care, like the early placement of feeding tubes, is crucial in the elderly population to give them the best chance of cure and survival or to provide the best palliation.

As discussed previously, adjuvant chemotherapy is often given in combination with radiation therapy to increase long-term survival following surgery. Sometimes 5-fluorouracil or Gemzar-based neoadjuvant chemotherapy, usually in combination with radiation therapy, is recommended before potentially curative surgery for pancreatic cancer. Only the most robust seniors are able to tolerate this type of intensive multi-modality therapy especially when Gemzar is used as the radio-sensitizing agent, and it is essential that you weigh the burdens and benefits of these aggressive approaches carefully. The additional benefit may only be marginal, and less aggressive approaches may be more appropriate.

Gemzar was approved by the Food and Drug Administration in 1996 for the palliative treatment of unresectable or metastatic pancreatic cancer. It is usually very well tolerated in this setting, and studies have shown that it may prolong survival. Perhaps more importantly, it often improves one's quality of life with respect to pain control, weight gain, and physical activity. Combination therapy with other anti-neoplastic agents (anticancer drugs) has not improved survival and is associated with an increased risk of side effects. However, pairing Gemzar with Tarceva, a targeted therapy discussed in Chapter 3, has provided a small survival benefit for patients with advanced or recurrent pancreatic cancer. It is generally well tolerated in older individuals. Xeloda (capecitabine) or 5-fluorouracil (5-FU) is used as a sensitizing agent with radiation therapy. Most older adults tolerate these regimens with minimal adverse events and equal benefit as compared with younger patients.

Though the side effects of cancer treatment are never less burdensome in the elderly, they can be managed by oncologists, especially geriatric oncologists, who work in teams with others who specialize in the care of the elderly. With appropriate care, healthy older patients do just as well with chemotherapy as do younger patients. Advances in supportive care, including antinausea medicines and medicines to increase red blood cells, have significantly decreased the side effects of chemotherapy and improved safety and the quality of life of individuals with pancreatic cancer. Nonetheless, there is risk especially if the patient is frail. The presence of severe comorbidities, age-related frailty, or underlying severe psychosocial problems may be obstacles for highly intensive treatment plans. Such patients may benefit from less complicated or potentially less toxic treatment plans.

COMMON TREATMENT COMPLICATIONS
IN THE ELDERLY

Anemia (low red blood cell count) is common in the elderly, especially the frail elderly. It decreases the effectiveness of chemotherapy and often causes fatigue, falls, cognitive decline (for example, dementia, disorientation, or confusion), and heart problems. Therefore, it is essential that anemia be recognized and corrected with red blood cell transfusions or the appropriate use of erythropoiesis-stimulating agents such as Procrit, Epogen (epoetin), or Aranesp (darbepoetin).

Myelosuppression (low white blood cell count) is also common in older patients getting chemotherapy or radiation therapy. Older patients with myelosuppression develop life-threatening infections more often than younger patients, and they may need to be treated in the hospital for many days. The liberal use of granulopoietic colony stimulating growth factors (or G-CSF, including Neupogen [filgrastim] and Neulasta [pegfilgrastim]) decreases the risk of infection, and makes it possible for older women to receive full doses of potentially curable adjuvant chemotherapy.

Thrombocytopenia (low platelet cell count in the blood) can cause serious bleeding problems. This is especially worrisome in an older person who is prone to falling. Someone who bleeds into the brain can suffer a serious and debilitating stroke. Like anemia and myelosuppression, thrombocytopenia is a side effect of many chemotherapy medicines (like Gemzar) and radiation therapy. It can usually be successfully managed by checking blood counts frequently and transfusing platelets when appropriate.

Mucositis (mouth sores) and diarrhea can cause severe dehydration in older patients who often are already dehydrated due to inadequate fluid intake and diuretics (water pills taken for high blood pressure or heart failure). Careful monitoring and the liberal use of drugs to treat diarrhea and oral and intravenous fluids are essential components of the management of older cancer patients, especially those receiving radiation, 5-FU, Xeloda, or combination chemotherapy and radiation therapy.

Kidney function declines as we age. Some of the medicines that older patients take to treat both their cancer- (for example, Gemzar, NSAIDs) and noncancer-related problems might make this worse. The dehydration that often accompanies cancer and its treatment can put additional stress on the kidneys. Fortunately, it is often possible to minimize these effects by carefully selecting and dosing appropriate drugs, managing polypharmacy, and preventing dehydration.

Neurotoxicity and cognitive effects (chemo brain) can be profoundly debilitating in patients who are already cognitively impaired (demented, disoriented, confused, etc.). Elderly patients with a history of falling, hearing loss or peripheral neuropathy (for example, nerve damage from diabetes) have decreased energy and are highly vulnerable to neurotoxic chemotherapy such as the taxanes or platinum compounds. Many of the medicines used to control nausea (antiemetics) or decrease the side effects of certain chemotherapy drugs are also potential neurotoxins. These include psychosis and agitation from Decadron (dexamethasone), agitation from Zantac, and sedation from Benadryl (diphenhydramine), and some of the antiemetics.

Fatigue is a near universal complaint of older cancer patients. It is particularly a problem for those who are socially isolated or depend upon others to help them with activities of daily living. It is not necessarily related to depression, but can be.

Depression is quite common in the elderly. In contrast to younger patients who often respond to a cancer diagnosis with anxiety, depression is the more common disorder in older cancer patients. With proper support and medical attention, many of these patients can safely receive anticancer treatment. Depression is also a common problem in people who have pancreatic cancer. If it requires treatment with antidepressant medicines, care should be taken in choosing an appropriate antidepressant (the SSRI category is often preferred) because many of these agents (in the tricyclic and MAO inhibitor categories) aggravate a number of medical problems that are common in older individuals, such as urinary retention related to an enlarged prostate, constipation, blurred vision, low blood pressure, rapid heart rate, and cognitive impairment.

Heart problems increase with age, and it is no surprise that older cancers patients have an increased risk of cardiac complications from surgery, radiation, and chemotherapy.

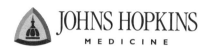

CHAPTER 11

TRUSTED RESOURCES—FINDING ADDITIONAL INFORMATION ABOUT PANCREATIC CANCER AND ITS TREATMENT

Your healthcare provider is the best source of information for questions and concerns regarding your diagnosis and treatment. Because no two patients are alike and recommendations can vary from one person to another depending on their personal circumstances, it is important to seek guidance from a provider who is familiar with your individual situation.

You can also get reliable information from the following sources.

American Cancer Society (ACS)

(800) ACS-2345 (227-2345)
http://www.cancer.org

The ACS is a nationwide, community-based voluntary health organization. You can find information and resources regarding pancreatic cancer.

American Pain Foundation (APF)
(888) 615-PAIN (615-7246)
http://www.painfoundation.org/about-apf/

The American Pain Foundation is an independent non-profit organization serving people with pain through information, advocacy, and support. The APF's mission is to improve the quality of life of people with pain by raising public awareness, providing practical information, promoting research, and advocating removing barriers and increasing access to effective pain management.

CancerCare, Inc.
(800) 813-HOPE (813-4673)
http://www.cancercare.org/
Email: info@cancercare.org

CancerCare is a national nonprofit organization that provides free, professional support services for anyone affected by cancer. Online and telephone patient and caregiver support groups are provided.

Cancer.Net
(888) 651-3038
http://www.cancer.net/portal/site/patient
Email: contactus@cancer.net

This is the official patient information Web site of the American Society of Clinical Oncology (ASCO). It provides information about pancreatic cancer.

CaringBridge
http://www.CaringBridge.org

CaringBridge offers free, personalized Web sites that allow people to stay in touch with family and friends during a health crisis, treatment, and recovery. Web sites provide a place to post journal entries and photos and to receive messages of hope and encouragement in a guestbook.

National Cancer Institute (NCI)

(800) 4-CANCER (422-6237, NCI's Cancer
Information Service)
http://www.cancer.gov/

The NCI offers educational information for pancreatic cancer patients and their family members. It also provides the latest information about available clinical trials. You can request free information by calling the toll-free number.

National Comprehensive Cancer Network (NCCN)

http://www.nccn.org/

The NCCN is an alliance of 21 of the world's leading cancer centers that are working together to develop treatment guidelines for most cancers and are dedicated to research that improves the quality, effectiveness, and efficiency of cancer care. NCCN offers a number of programs to help you and your family make informed decisions about your health.

National Pancreas Foundation

(866) 726-2737
http://www.pancreasfoundation.org/

The National Pancreas Foundation supports research of diseases of the pancreas and provides information and humanitarian services to those people who are suffering from such diseases.

OncoLink

http://www.oncolink.org/

OncoLink is a Web site that provides the latest news on cancer treatment, cancer research, oncology advances, and cancer clinical trials.

Pancreatic Cancer Action Network (PanCAN)

(877) 272-6226

http://www.pancan.org/

PanCAN provides patient services, community outreach, and education; works to generate public policy; and supplies funding for research support. It provides extensive information about pancreatic cancer, including treatment options, clinical trials, specialists, support groups, and diet and nutrition. PanCAN's Patient and Liaison Services (PALS) is a source of quality education and resources for pancreatic cancer patients, families, and health professionals. It is a comprehensive, free, call-in information program that matches trained, dedicated PALS associates one-on-one with callers.

Pancreatica

(831) 658-0600

http://www.pancreatica.org/

This Web site serves as a worldwide gathering point on the Internet for the latest news and information regarding clinical trials and other responsible medical care in the treatment of pancreatic cancer.

Well Spouse Association

http://www.wellspouse.org

Well Spouse Association is a national organization focusing exclusively on the needs of all spouses caring for a chronically ill or disabled husband, wife, or partner.

WHERE CAN I GET HELP WITH FINANCIAL OR LEGAL CONCERNS?

Accompanying any serious illness are questions and concerns related to expenses incurred as a result of treatment, health insurance coverage, and legal issues related to employment or financial matters. The following is a list of national resources to aid you in addressing these types of concerns.

National Coalition for Cancer Survivorship (NCCS)

(888) 650-9127
(877) NCCS-YES (622-7937, for the Cancer Survival Toolbox)
http://www.canceradvocacy.org
Email: info@canceradvocacy.org

This network of independent groups and individuals provides information and resources about cancer support, advocacy, and quality-of-life issues. NCCS also helps cancer patients deal with insurance or job discrimination and other related legal matters.

Patient Advocate Foundation

(800) 532-5274
http://www.patientadvocate.org
Email: help@patientadvocate.org

This organization provides educational information about managed care, insurance issues, and legal counseling on debt intervention, job discrimination issues, and insurance denials of coverage.

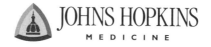

INFORMATION ABOUT
JOHNS HOPKINS

Pancreas Multidisciplinary Cancer Clinic at Johns Hopkins
Appointment Line: (410) 933-PANC (933-7262)
or (410) 955-5718
http://pathology.jhu.edu/pancreas/MDC/index.php

The Pancreas Multidisciplinary Cancer Clinic is a part of the Sidney Kimmel Comprehensive Cancer Center at Johns Hopkins where the goal is to provide the highest quality of care to patients with pancreatic cancer. The clinic is designed to evaluate patients with known or suspected pancreatic cancer. The clinic is committed to a single-day comprehensive evaluation of a patient incorporating all the resources available for the education, diagnosis, treatment, and research of pancreatic cancer by some of the top pancreatic cancer clinicians and specialists in the country. Patients have access to state of the art radiologic imaging and expert radiologists and leading pancreas pathologists, as well as the latest and most promising antineoplastic and radiation therapies. A diagnosis of pancreatic cancer can be stressful and overwhelming. All members of the Pancreas Multidisciplinary Cancer Clinic are dedicated to assisting patients and caregivers.

Johns Hopkins Hospital Department of Surgery
New Patient Referral

Appointment Line: (410) 933-1233

Patients have access to surgeons with vast experience in performing a full range of surgical treatments for pancreatic surgery, including minimally invasive approaches. Surgeons at Johns Hopkins have performed over 3,000 Whipple resections, more than any other institution in the world. A number of studies have shown that surgical volume (the number of pancreatic resections a center performs each year) is a strong predictor of patient outcome. In 2002, a study in the *New England Journal of Medicine* by Dr. Birkmeyer and colleagues from Vermont's Department of Veteran Affairs reported that the mortality rate for Whipple procedures at low-volume centers was 16.3%, while the mortality rate for the same surgery at high-volume centers was only 3.8%. From their analyses the authors conclude that patients "can significantly reduce their risk of operative death by selecting a high-volume hospital." (*N Engl J Med.* 2002;346(15):1128–1137). High-volume centers were defined in this study as centers that perform more than 16 Whipple procedures per year. More than 200 Whipple procedures are performed at Johns Hopkins Hospital each year, and the mortality rate is less than 2%.

About the Sidney Kimmel Comprehensive
Cancer Center at Johns Hopkins

http://www.hopkinskimmelcancercenter.org

Since its inception in 1973, the Sidney Kimmel Comprehensive Cancer Center at Johns Hopkins has been dedicated to better understanding human cancers and finding more effective treatments. One of only 40 cancer centers in the country designated by the National Cancer Institute (http://www.cancer.gov) as a Comprehensive Cancer Center, the Johns Hopkins Kimmel Cancer Center has active programs in clinical research, laboratory research, education, community outreach, and prevention and control, and is the only Comprehensive Cancer Center in the state of Maryland.

About Johns Hopkins Medicine

http://www.hopkinsmedicine.org

Johns Hopkins Medicine unites physicians and scientists of the Johns Hopkins University School of Medicine with the organizations, health professionals, and facilities of the Johns Hopkins Health System. Its mission is to improve the health of the community and the world by setting the standard of excellence in medical education, research, and clinical care. Diverse and inclusive, Johns Hopkins Medicine has provided international leadership in the education of physicians and medical scientists in biomedical research and in the application of medical knowledge to sustain health since The Johns Hopkins Hospital opened in 1889.

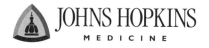

FURTHER READING

100 *Questions & Answers About Pancreatic Cancer, Second Edition,* Eileen O'Reilly, MD, and Joanne Frankel Kelvin, RN, MSN, Jones and Bartlett Publishers, 2010.

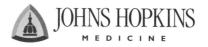

GLOSSARY

Adjuvant therapy: Treatment given after the primary treatment to increase the chances of cure, and treatment to prevent the cancer from recurring, such as chemotherapy and radiation therapy.

Advance directives: Legal documents that allow people to express their decisions regarding what they do and don't want to have done during their last weeks or months in case they become unable to communicate effectively.

Advanced practice nurse: A registered nurse with advanced training, education, knowledge, and skills. These nurses have a Master's degree or a doctorate.

Alternative therapy: A treatment that has not been tested scientifically and is used in place of traditional treatments, such as herbals.

Americans with Disabilities Act (ADA): Enacted in 1990, the ADA prohibits discrimination because of disability. The Act defines disability as "a physical or mental impairment that substantially limits one or more major life activities."

Anemia: An abnormally low number of red blood cells circulating in the body that may be due to bleeding or lack of blood production by the bone marrow. It may also be a side effect of treatment or malnutrition.

Anesthesia pain physician: An anesthesiologist who specialized in the treatment of pain using both medicines and special procedures such as nerve blocks.

Anesthesiologist: A doctor who specializes in putting people to sleep using anesthesia in the operating room.

Antineoplastic: Drugs that fight the growth of cancer cells, also called anticancer drugs or chemotherapy.

Ascites: Build-up of fluid in the space between the tissues lining the abdomen and the abdominal organs. These are generally related to liver failure from cancer that is taking over the liver.

Biopsy: A procedure in which cells are collected for microscopic examination.

Brain fog: A common side effect of taking drugs that fight cancer, but also affect the brain causing temporary problems with memory and concentration. Also known as chemo brain.

Cancer: The presence of malignant cells.

Carbohydrate antigen 19-9 (CA 19-9): This is a tumor marker for pancreatic cancer and is most useful as a surveillance marker after the diagnosis of pancreatic cancer is confirmed.

Carcinoembryonic antigen (CEA): This is used as a tumor marker in many gastrointestinal cancers.

Carcinomas: Cancers that form in the surface cells of different tissues.

Celiac axis: Major blood vessels that supply blood to the stomach, liver, and spleen.

Cell proliferation: Rapid growth and reproduction of cells.

Cells: Basic elements of tissues. The appearance and composition of individual cells are unique to the tissue they compose.

Chemotherapy: The use of chemical agents (drugs) to treat cancer cells that may be found anywhere in the body.

Chemotherapy regimen: The schedule and dosage of chemotherapy drugs to treat a cancer.

Chronic pain: Pain that is present for long periods of time, though not always at the same intensity.

Clinical trial: A study of a drug or treatment with a large group of people testing the treatment.

Complementary therapy: Therapy that is added to conventional or traditional treatments. Complementary therapy may ease the side effects of standard treatments or provide physical or mental benefits to patients with cancer. Examples include massage therapy to relieve stress and acupuncture to relieve pain or nausea.

Cumulative: Keep adding on.

Deep vein thrombosis: Formation of a thrombus (blood clot) in the leg or pelvis. A deep vein thrombosis can also occur in the arm.

Dehydration: Dryness resulting from the removal of water or the depletion of bodily fluids.

Delayed gastric emptying (DGE): Inability of the stomach to empty its contents without evidence of a blockage or obstruction.

Dietician: A food and nutrition expert.

Drains: Tubes that may be placed at the time of surgery to drain extra fluid from the remaining pancreas or around the bile duct. Patients sometimes go home with the drains.

Durable power of attorney: Allows a specific family member to legally make all your decisions, personal and financial, in case you become incapacitated.

Endocrinologist: A specialist that treats endocrine system disorders including diabetes, hyperthyroidism, and many other hormone imbalances.

Endoscopic retrograde cholangiopancreatography (ERCP): A test that may be used to help delineate the cause of an obstruction and allow placement of a stent to treat the jaundice caused by the obstruction.

Endoscopic ultrasound (EUS): A test sometimes used to diagnose pancreatic cancer. An EUS may help to determine the size and location of the tumor in the pancreas, and if the tumor has spread to nearby lymph nodes, blood vessels, or other tissues.

Endoscopist: A doctor (gastroenterologist) who specializes in performing studies that look at the inside of the gastrointestinal tract using flexible cameras.

Endoscopy: Looking inside the body for medical reasons using an endoscope, which is an instrument used to examine the interior of a hollow organ or cavity of the body.

Enzymes: Substances that break down carbohydrates, proteins, and fats for digestion and absorption. Digestive enzymes made by the pancreas include lipase to break down fats, amylase to break down sugars and carbohydrates, and protease to break down proteins.

Fine needle aspiration (FNA): A way to biopsy pancreatic masses using a very thin needle to collect fluid or cells directly from the pancreas mass. Physicians can then look at the cells under a microscope to see if they are cancerous.

Gastric outlet obstruction: Blockage of the stomach from tumor.

Gastrointestinal (GI) symptoms: Common medical conditions that include stomach pain, heartburn, diarrhea, constipation, nausea, and vomiting.

Grade: Describes how quickly the cancer is growing based on the appearance of the cells under the microscope.

Healthcare proxy: Permits a designated person to make decisions regarding your medical treatment when you are unable to do so.

Immune system: Complex network of tissues, organs, cells, and chemicals that protects the body from infection and illness.

In situ: A cancer that is still in place (noninvasive) or has no potential of spreading to another organ.

Informed consent: A process by which patients participating in a clinical study are provided with all available information regarding the experimental treatment prior to consenting to receive that treatment. Informed consents are also obtained for any invasive procedure or surgery.

Intraoperative brachytherapy: Radiation therapy given in the operating room at the time of surgery.

Intraoperative radiation therapy: Radiation therapy given in the operating room at the time of surgery.

Invasive cancer: Cancer that has the potential to spread, or metastasize, to other organs such as the liver. Most pancreatic cancers are invasive.

Jaundice: Yellowish coloring of the skin and sclerae (whites) of the eyes usually caused by an increase in bilirubin in the blood.

Laparoscopy: Surgery that uses a thin, lighted tube, or laparoscope, with a camera inserted through an incision in the belly to look at the abdominal organs.

Living will: Outlines what care you want in the event you become unable to communicate due to coma or heavy sedation.

Lymph nodes: Tissues in the lymphatic system that filter lymph fluid and help the immune system fight disease. Cancer can spread from the pancreas to other organs through the lymph nodes.

Malabsorption: Difficulty digesting or absorbing nutrients from food into the bloodstream, which can cause diarrhea.

Malnutrition: A condition that develops when the body does not get the right amount of the vitamins, minerals, and other nutrients it needs to maintain healthy tissues and organ function.

Medical oncologist: *See* oncologist.

Mental health counselor: A trained professional that counsels families, individuals, groups, and couples to promote optimal mental health and well being.

Metastasis, metastasize: The spread of cancer to other organ sites, such as the liver.

Mortality: The statistical calculation of death rates due to a specific disease within a population.

Mutation: A gene with a mistake or alteration in its DNA sequence.

Nasogastric tube: A tube that runs from the nose into the stomach to help empty the stomach. Nasogastric tubes are often placed at the time of surgery.

Neoadjuvant therapy: Therapy that is started before the primary treatment.

Noninvasive cancer: Cancer that is confined to tissue of origin and has no potential to spread to distant organs.

Obstructive jaundice: Tumor blocking the bile duct where it enters the pancreas that results in yellow coloring of the eyes and skin.

Oncologist: A cancer specialist who helps determine treatment choices.

Opioids: Medicines derived from morphine and similar chemicals.

Palliative care: Care to relieve the symptoms of cancer and to keep the best quality of life for as long as possible without seeking to cure cancer.

Pancreas leak: Leakage of contents from the pancreas gland after surgery. The pancreas has powerful digestive enzymes and as these enzymes leak, an abdominal infection can result.

Pathologist: A specialist trained to distinguish normal from abnormal cells.

Percutaneous biliary drain (PBD): A tube that is placed into the liver and then threaded into the major bile duct that travels to the back side of the pancreas and finally empties into the first part of the small bowel (duodenum).

Percutaneous transhepatic cholangiogram (PTC): A procedure in which a special X-ray takes pictures of the bile ducts that drain the liver.

Peripheral neuropathy: A problem with the nerves that carry information to and from the brain and spinal cord. This can produce pain, loss of sensation, and an inability to control muscles.

Positron Emission Tomography (PET) scan: A special scan using radioactive glucose (sugar) to look and see if the cancer has spread or metastasized.

Prognosis: An estimation of the likely outcome of an illness based upon the patient's current status and the available treatments.

Protocols: The research plan for how a drug is given and to whom it is given.

Pruritus: A sensation that causes one to scratch. More commonly known as itchiness.

Psychologist: A doctor that studies the mind and behavior of humans.

Pulmonary embolism: A blood clot in the lungs.

Radiation oncologist: A doctor who specializes in giving radiation to treat cancer.

Radiation therapy: Use of high-energy X-rays to kill cancer cells and shrink tumors.

Radiologist: A doctor who reads X-ray studies, including CT scans.

Red blood cells (RBC): Cells in the blood whose primary function is carrying oxygen to tissues.

Risk factors: Any factors that contribute to an increased possibility of getting cancer.

Sex therapist: May be a psychiatrist, a marriage and family therapist, a psychologist, or a clinical social worker that is specially trained in sex therapy. A sex therapist assists those persons experiencing problems with sexual issues to overcome them and to regain an active sex life.

Stage: A numerical determination of how far the cancer has progressed.

Steatorrhea: Presence of an excessive amount of fat in the stool. Stools may float due to excess lipid, have an oily appearance, and be especially foul smelling.

Stent: A small straw-like tube used to bypass a blockage.

Stimulant: Chemical substances that cause temporary improvements in either mental or physical function or both. Examples of these kinds of effects include enhanced alertness and wakefulness.

Superior mesenteric artery: A major blood vessel that is found behind the pancreas and supplies blood to all the small intestines.

Superior mesenteric vein: A major blood vessel that is found behind the pancreas and next to the superior mesenteric artery. The superior mesenteric vein drains blood from the small intestines.

Supportive therapy: Any form of treatment intended to relieve symptoms or help the patient live with them.

Surgical oncologist: A surgeon who specializes in cancer surgery.

Systemic treatment: Treatment that goes to all parts of the body.

Targeted therapy: Treatment that targets specific molecules involved in carcinogenesis or tumor growth.

Toxin: A poisonous substance that can be anywhere from acutely dangerous to immediately fatal.

Whipple procedure: A surgical operation to remove pancreatic cancer, also known as a pancreaticoduodenectomy.

INDEX

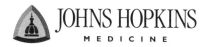

INDEX